Testosterone

A Guide to More Muscle and Upgraded Living

(How to Boost Testosterone Naturally and Feel Amazing)

Shelly Garcia

Published By **Darby Connor**

Shelly Garcia

All Rights Reserved

Testosterone: A Guide to More Muscle and Upgraded Living (How to Boost Testosterone Naturally and Feel Amazing)

ISBN   978-1-77485-813-4

No part of this guidebook shall be reproduced in any form without permission in writing from the publisher except in the case of brief quotations embodied in critical articles or reviews.

Legal & Disclaimer

The information contained in this ebook is not designed to replace or take the place of any form of medicine or professional medical advice. The information in this ebook has been provided for educational & entertainment purposes only.

The information contained in this book has been compiled from sources deemed reliable, and it is accurate to the best of the Author's knowledge; however, the Author cannot guarantee its accuracy and validity and cannot be held liable for any errors or omissions. Changes are periodically made to this book. You must consult your doctor or get professional medical advice before using any of the suggested remedies, techniques, or information in this book.

Upon using the information contained in this book, you agree to hold harmless the Author from and against any damages, costs, and expenses, including any legal fees potentially resulting from the application of any of the information provided by this guide. This disclaimer applies to any damages or injury caused by the use and application, whether directly or indirectly, of any advice or information presented, whether for breach of contract, tort, negligence, personal injury, criminal intent, or under any other cause of action.

You agree to accept all risks of using the information presented inside this book. You need to consult a professional medical practitioner in order to ensure you are both able and healthy enough to participate in this program.

TABLE OF CONTENTS

Introduction 1

Chapter 1: Inflluence Of Testosterone 8

Chapter 2: What's Causing My Low
Testosterone? 25

Chapter 3: Rise Testosterone By
Consuming More Nutrients.................... 35

Chapter 4: Essential Supplements.......... 50

Chapter 5: Testosterone Training Guide 63

Chapter 6: Life Style And Behavioral
Modifications.. 69

Chapter 7: What Should I Know To Be
Aware Of Regarding Your Testosterone
Level?.. 75

Chapter 8: Essentials For Low Testosterone
Levels As Well As Testosterone
Replacement Therapy 101

Chapter 9: What Testosterone Is Vital? 145

Conclusion 182

Introduction

Testosterone is the main and possibly the most vital male hormone that men produce. It is released by testes in male mammals , and in a lesser degree by adrenal glands. Testosterone is a class of male hormones referred to as anabolic steroids or androgens. It is interesting to note that testosterone is secreted and produced by females. It is found in their bloodstreams and is created by the ovaries and the adrenal glands. There is however an enormous and substantial variation in the amounts of testosterone present in the blood of a man as compared to females. Males have twenty times the testosterone of women.

Because it is mostly male-specific this is logical to make this huge distinction. Testosterone is the hormone that is responsible in promoting the growth of male characteristics prior to birth, and for influencing secondary male characteristics that develop during puberty.

Different types of Testosterone

The scientifically speaking there are three types of testosterone throughout the bloodstream. They are Free testosterone, SHBG-bound testosterone, and albumin-bound testosterone. This is the distinction between the three different forms of testosterone hormone.

Sex Hormone Binding Globulin (SHBG) is an glycoprotein that bonds itself to sexual hormones. In this instance, it bonds its self to testosterone. The bond is typically strong, and makes the testosterone molecule that is bound to it to be biologically inert. It actually blocks the function in the testosterone molecule. SHBG is created by the liver and helps to regulate the amount and quantity of testosterone in the blood stream.

albumin bound testosterone. In this situation there is a lower percentage of testosterone is linked by serum albumin. Serum albumin is a common blood component. The bond created between the albumin and testosterone molecule is extremely fragile. Sometimes this group isn't ever considered to be to be bound at all. If this bond breaks the release of more testosterone into the bloodstream. In a testosterone test several labs will categorize albumin bound testosterone as well as free testosterone as one.

Free testosterone is the term used to describe testosterone molecules, which are unbound and not bound. It's typically a small proportion of the secreted testosterone (1-2 percent). The testosterone is in its pure form with no connected protein molecules. Being biologically active means that testosterone molecules can be absorbed into cells of the body, trigger receptors, and cause an effect of testosterone on the mind and body.

Production of Testosterone

As mentioned earlier testosterone is made in the male human body through two organs: testosterone glands in the adrenals as well as testes. The majority of testosterone is produced by the testes. This makes up more than 90% of the testosterone that is produced. The process of making testosterone is extremely complex and is a complex process that involves many other hormones, in addition to the pituitary gland, the hypothalamus gland, and of course the testicles. This is the way it works.

All of it begins with the brain. The hypothalamus, an area that is located in the brain is able to detect that the body is lacking levels of testosterone and needs more. It secretes gonadotropin-releasing hormone, which is the signal that is sent to yet another important gland located at the base of the brain. This is the pituitary .

The pituitary gland functions as an endocrine gland. Its hormones that it releases are absorbed directly into the blood stream and rather than through an artery or a vessel. Once the pituitary gland detects the gonadotropin-releasing hormone from the hypothalamus, it kick-starts its own production of two vital hormones.

The hormones involved include Luteinizing Hormone (LH) and Follicle Stimulating Hormone (FSH). Both hormones are transported directly from the bloodstream to the testicles.

Humans are blessed with testes external to them which are located within the scrotum. It is a double suspended sack which houses the tests. After these two hormones that are released from the pituitary gland enter the testicles, two important actions are initiated by these hormones.

The FSH initiates an opportunistic process called spermatogenesis that is, the production of sperm. In contrast LH LH stimulates a specific group of cells that are specialized (found within the testes) also known as Leydig cells to make testosterone.

The leydig-cells create testosterone by an extremely complex process that involves the conversion cholesterol into testosterone hormone. This cholesterol is the primary building block of testosterone.

What is happening is that in when there is LH the function of cholesterol desmolase is dramatically elevated. Cholesterol desmolase enzyme responsible for catalyzing the process making cholesterol into pregnenolone.

It is because of this process that the Leydig-cells become capable of synthesizing and secreting testosterone into bloodstream.

When blood is circulated there is a higher percentage of testosterone is attached to albumin molecules or SHBG. They are biologically inert.

The rest is testosterone free that is not bound or biologically active.

Regulation and Control of Testosterone Regulation of Testosterone

As with all processes within the body there exists an optimal amount that should be maintained. This avoids the possibility of excessive or insufficient testosterone production. The production of testosterone and its release into the bloodstream is again determined by the hypothalamus as well as the pituitary gland.

After production of testosterone and release into the blood stream, the hypothalamus detects this surge in testosterone and it suppresses the production of gonadotropin-releasing hormone.

This is an indication for the pituitary gland that it needs to lower the manufacturing of LH as well as FSH. This means that fewer of these hormones reach the testicles, and consequently testosterone production decreases.

As levels of testosterone begin to fall, negative feedback also falls and the hypothalamus goes back to secreting gonadotropin-releasing hormone. The whole cycle of production of testosterone is over.

It's a continuous cycle that makes sure the body has enough testosterone to meet its requirements. It helps keep testosterone levels in the blood under control extremely efficiently.

Androgens generally play two distinct functions that they play in the male body. One is to trigger the anabolic effects, and the second one is to trigger the androgenic impact. The anabolic effects of androgens are the growth of muscle mass and stronger. Androgenic results are more involved regarding sexual growth. These effects include maturation of the sex organs as well as voice development and beard growth , among other secondary sexual traits.

Chapter 1: Inflluence Of Testosterone

Testosterone is a powerful male hormone that has confirmed to be the primary factor involved in its development into a broad assortment of male traits. In essence, of the hormones that are androgenic testosterone is the most important.

The production begins just seven weeks of conception. Its rates significantly increase during puberty, and highest in late teens. Below is a glimpse into this aspect.

The majority of men have adequate levels of this hormone however, it is not uncommon for people to have lower than the recommended levels due to various reasons. This is usually the cause of the medical condition called hypogonadism. The effect of testosterone in men is broad, and it could influence the health and functioning of various systems. This article is designed to provide a detailed explanation of the most prominent results of testosterone in males.

Testosterone & endocrine system

The endocrine system comprises of several glands, whose main function is to synthesize various hormones your body needs. One of them is the pituitary gland that plays a role in the production of testosterone.

The hypothalamus located within the brain usually informs the gland about the amount of testosterone the body requires. Once this is done the pituitary gland sends the right message to the testes that are the primary source of testosterone. This is usually the case for the development of male traits in the period of adolescence.

Testosterone & reproduction system

As mentioned earlier testosterone production is triggered about 7 weeks following fertilization of the egg. In this period, the hormone plays an important part in the growth of male sexual organs. Then, during puberty it encourages the growth of the testicles and penis. It also contributes to making sperm production on a regular basis. The men who have lower levels of testosterone are characterized by having lower sexual desire. A drastic drop in levels of testosterone can be caused by an extended absence from sexual activities. Most of the time, this causes male health issues like impermanence

Testosterone & central nervous system

The impact of testosterone is experienced by the central nervous system, and it is a key factor in the formation of behavioral traits like aggressiveness and dominant. The proper levels of this hormone can boost competitiveness as in boosting self-esteem.

People who are involved in intensely athletic activities are said to have high amounts of testosterone. However people with low levels are usually associated with lower confidence levels and sometimes, even a lack of motivation. The lower concentrations of testosterone have been associated with problems with concentration as well as melancholia. It can also negatively impact sleep.

Testosterone & kidneys

The effects of testosterone can be extended to the functioning in the kidneys. This hormone has been found to affect the kidney hormone known as erythropoietin. This hormone helps in stimulating the production of red blood cells inside the bone marrow. Insufficient levels of testosterone could cause anemia.

Testosterone, muscles and bones

Testosterone is, by far, the most important element in the proper development of muscle mass and strength. In this regard it acts by altering neurotransmitters that are found in the brain that increase the size of tissue for males.

This hormone also functions through DNA receptors, which encourage the production of more protein. In addition, they it plays a major part in boosting levels of human growth hormone in the body. This enables the rapid development of muscle mass when a male body is exposed to an appropriate workout routine. Testosterone also is known to play an important role in maintaining bone density. The hormone's levels are low and are associated to bone fractures and breakage.

Testosterone and hair and skin

The effects of testosterone can be linked to the transition from childhood into adulthood for males. This hormone plays a role in promoting growth of body hair, facial hair, and pubic hair. In terms of our skins, testosterone is believed to be an amazing sun-protection for males.

This hormone also stimulates the growth of collagen and elastin networks that can result in a more sturdier skin, especially in comparison to females.

Testosterone & brain

Testosterone is also known to have a wide-ranging effect in the mind. Although the field of research is still relatively new and the results seem to be contradictory however, there is a consensus that high levels of the hormone are believed to greatly enhance cognitive performance. This naturally includes memory, attention span and even spatial vision capabilities.

A new study has shown that low levels of testosterone are a cause of poor performance on cognitive tests in men. Furthermore, it has been found that men with lower levels of testosterone are susceptible to cognitive decline.

In the extreme they can develop conditions like dementia or Alzheimer's disease. The latter is frequent for older men, who's testosterone production is in lower levels.

Testosterone & sex drive

The effects of testosterone has a significant impact on libido, both women and men. For males specifically, extensive research has revealed that testosterone plays an important role in the desire to have sexual intimacy, and eventually performance.

The men who have lower level of testosterone frequently recognized for their inability to get a good sexual relations. This is in addition to the possibility of getting an erection that is hard and having an intense gasp.

However those who have sufficient amounts of the hormone said to be unaffected in this regard and can be satisfied with their spouses as well as themselves relaxed way.

The significance of TESTOSTERONE

Mental Concentration

Unfortunately, a lot of the time when people are thinking about testosterone's capabilities but they do not think about its impact on cognitive processes.

However, based on a variety of studies, it has been determined that testosterone levels do influence cognitive processes and, consequently, can affect the mental performance of men.

Of all the functions of the brain memory is the most delicate. Based on the research that were conducted, it was found out that as we advances in age, learning slows down, and information that is new takes longer to process.

Testosterone levels decrease as age increases. After experimenting with different methods researchers discovered that testosterone increases synaptic plasticity which, in turn, improves memory.

Testosterone levels are also related to mood. One benefit of having high levels of testosterone is the ability to maintain an enlightened and positive mood all the time. The low level of testosterone can lead to an uneasy state as people become quiet and silent.

Muscle mass increases

It is a fact that bodybuilders increase their testosterone levels in a controlled manner. The reason for this is they want to build masses; Unfortunately, a lot of them get themselves overdone, with the which results in an increase in deformation.

The benefit of having high T levels are that the body's muscular mass will increase to a high level, While low levels of T could result in shrinking of muscles and generally sagging the body.

Heart Healthy Heart

T levels are also connected to heart problems. According to scientists, both high and low T levels could be fatal. They could increase the risk of developing heart diseases or influence how your heart operates. In this way, the right T levels can drastically lower the risk of suffering from cardiac-related illnesses such as peripheral artery diseases. T levels, particularly when they are high, are believed to cause an increase in cholesterol levels in the blood vessels which deliver vital blood flow to the heart. It could lead to heart attacks. In the end, having optimal concentrations of T are the best method of reducing the risk of heart issues.

Strong Erection

Although the erection process is definitely an androgen-dependent process, testosterone are still are a factor in erection, as low T levels have been shown to be the cause of Erectile Dysfunction. However, the question is at what point does the person begin experiencing ED. To investigate this possibility studies were conducted on males with obvious hypogonadism. It was found that a decrease in frequency, rigidity, and frequency of erections were a regular characteristic of all.

According to research that normal adults don't need testosterone to allow normal erections to occur. Therefore, if testosterone levels that are optimal are the main ingredient. the increase in levels doesn't add nothing to the frequency or intensity of an erection.

Healthy Libido

In the case of male libido and sexual desire, testosterone is an important part. Contrary to erection in which when the ideal level has been attained, no changes are observed when the levels rise, in the libido process, there's an extremely fine line.

The men with the highest levels of testosterone have a healthy libido that is not low or high. If testosterone levels exceed normal range, the person becomes unpredictable; they may have an extremely strong sex drive, but occasionally they appear normal. When T is low sexual drive is extremely low and in some cases, libido disappears completely.

Strong Bones

As people get older, their levels of T decrease, which leads to a decrease in bone density. This may result in osteoporosis. It is a common occurrence for older people, they are sometimes advised to undergo T treatment where Testosterone hormones are created within their bodies by artificial means. A healthy level of T is essential to a healthy and perfect bone density by increasing its volume and mass and consequently results in not only more robust, but also healthier bones but also healthier ones.

Plenty of Energy

As we mentioned previously One of the most common signs that are associated with testosterone deficiency is the chronic fatigue. When levels drop to low, the person becomes weak and tired quickly. Achieving optimal levels as well as greater levels help one become stronger and better. When T levels are low the exercise and training process becomes tiring.

But, when you have the right levels of T you will have a great deal of energy and remains active throughout. Energy is vital because it keeps your body active, promotes a healthy metabolism, and improves the level of alertness throughout the day. In short high levels of T help can make you productive and generally robust.

Reduced body fat

Since T levels are connected to muscle growth and the results are contingent on the level, and low T levels could cause your body to shrink, while high T levels could result in the development of deformities. The optimal levels of T however are believed to promote the growth of healthy muscles.

Body fats decrease automatically as muscle buildup increases and, as such, the optimal levels of T help to burn the fat in your body and reduces the possibility of being afflicted by excess fat-related illnesses like weight gain. However, it is important to be aware of not exceeding the thresholds that are ideal, your body's cholesterol levels start to increase in arteries.

Athletic Performance

Testosterone levels can be linked to vitality, alertness, and strength. A healthy T level keeps you in constant motion and, as a result, allows the person more competitive in the sport they play. Many people know that the majority of athletes dope.

Doping typically involves the use of substances which increase your activeness and encourage the production of testosterone. If you are found to be doing this you'll be punished and therefore you shouldn't ever think about it. You can still improve your performance in athletics with the right T levels, it is important to maintain it.

A symptom that indicates your TESTOSTERONE is decreasing.

The difficulty in getting an sexual erection

As we will see, testosterone acts as the hormone that is required to increase a man's sexual desire. This hormone permits the person to have an sexual erection. However, it's important to remember that testosterone by itself will make an erection happen in the first place, but it will stimulate certain receptor cells within the brain that generate nitric Oxide. This is the nitric acid which causes an erection.

If a person has testosterone levels that are low it is possible that he will have difficulty getting an erection after an affair. In other instances, he might have erections that occur spontaneously, such as in the night. It is vital to know that there are a variety of other medical conditions that might hinder the process of erection which is why it's crucial to perform tests to determine if it's the T levels that are bringing symptoms.

Low Sex Drive

Testosterone plays a role in the libido of both genders. It is common for males to feel less sexual desire as they age. If the reduction in sex drive is severe, it could be an indication of low levels of testosterone.

If T levels are low the male is unlikely to have an erection, and if there is one, it will not be enough to allow the man to be able to participate in an intimate relationship. A low T level can reduce libido among women, as well as other issues like mood swings as well as hormonal fluctuations.

Semen is reduced

Semen is the milky liquid which helps in the mobility of the sperms. Testosterone is the hormone that is needed for producing this type of fluid. This means that the greater the amount of semen a person is able to produce in the body,, the more semen he produces. If a person has an insufficient amount of semen will see a decrease in the amount of semen they produce when they ejaculate.

Muscle mass is reduced

Testosterone plays a role in the building and strengthening of muscles. People with low levels of T are likely to experience a decrease in strength and mass. If you struggle to reverse muscle loss through physical exercises, like weight training, will be unable to recover the muscles they lost.

Hair loss

Testosterone is a key component in many body functions, including for the creation of hair. As we've seen hair loss is a normal problem for men particularly as they get older. Men with low testosterone levels might suffer from hair loss in different areas of the body like facial hair.

Fatigue and lack of energy

Men with low levels of testosterone will feel tired and often feel tired. If you are constantly exhausted even in bed it is time to test to determine your testosterone level. If you have low testosterone levels, levels may also be unable to exercise since they constantly complain about being exhausted. When they engage in sport, those who have low levels of T get exhausted and tired. They also spend a lot of time.

Body fat is increased

The testosterone level within the body decreases and the body begins to boost the amount of estrogen produced. The most embarrassing thing happens when a person is affected by large male breasts. It is imperative to remember that there are estrogens that are beneficial as well as the best ones. The higher levels of estradiol and prolactin are able to feminize male body. However, the right estrogens can assist in the prevention of heart-related diseases. Certain estrogens are also connected to the development of prostate tumors.

Reduced bone mass

The low levels of testosterone have been linked to a condition called osteoporosis . It is the bone loss. Osteoporosis tends to be suffered by women. But men with low testosterone levels could also face the same problem. We have mentioned before testosterone plays a role in strengthening bones. People with low testosterone levels are more prone to fractures of bones.

Changes in mood

It is normal that women experience changes in their mood because estrogen levels decrease in menses. It's the same scenario that men experience when testosterone levels drop and testosterone can affect mental health and mood. Many studies have shown that people who have lower levels of this hormone are more likely to suffer from less focus, which can make people more irritable.

Testicles shrieking

The men who have very low testosterone levels could notice a decrease in the dimensions of the testicle. The testicles could appear less firm than they usually do.

A decrease in sensitivity in the genital area (genital numbness)

If the testosterone levels are low, males may feel less sensitive to their genital regions. A few may experience an numbness in the same area. It is crucial to remember that testosterone levels diminish naturally as you get older. People will experience different levels of these signs. If you are experiencing any of these symptoms it is recommended that you spoke to your physician who will perform tests to determine whether you suffer from an issue with your T levels.

Chapter 2: What's Causing My Low

Testosterone?

As we've mentioned before testosterone plays a significant influence on our mind as well as body and sexual functions. The reason for low testosterone in men could be attributed to routines or bad habits. routines we engage in every day can cause low testosterone levels and at times, we don't realize that we are harming our bodies. Let's look at some of the most prevalent reasons:

Obesity: Testosterone converts into estrogen by men naturally. It is the production of estrogen that can help men maintain a healthy bone density. But, if a person is obese or overweight, it is believed that the transformation of testosterone into estrogen is mainly triggered in fat cells.

Due to the presence of fat cells within our bodies, more testosterone is transformed into estrogen, which causes lower levels of testosterone. Furthermore, being overweight is often associated with a variety of ailments (type two diabetes, or hypertension) that are associated with low testosterone levels.

Stress: The ability to reproduce of males is diminished when they are continuously under stress. The stress that is constant increases cortisol levels and reduces the Central hormone channels. In turn, the secretion of hormones that regulate reproduction as well as testosterone production is reduced. Furthermore, stress hinders testosterone from exerting a positive influence upon the body.

Excessive alcohol consumption: Drinking, even two drinks in a day, could lead to lower testosterone levels of 6-8 percent for men. Hops (an ingredient used in the production of beer) possess estrogen-like properties that negatively affect testosterone.

Sugar intake: Consuming sugar food items (candy cookies, cookies, bread or soda) raise blood glucose levels that increases the production of insulin by the pancreas. In the wake of increased insulin levels, the central hormone pathway within the body gets affected, resulting in decreased testosterone production.

BPA in plastic: BPA is synthetic chemical; Bisphenol - A found in a variety of plastic containers, it releases when heated. The people who are exposed to BPA have low T levels and may also have fertility issues. Because BPA is among the most significant factors that result in low testosterone, it's suggested to drink water from glass or stainless steel bottles rather than plastic bottles.

Lack of sleep Because of the demands of modern life sleep deprivation is one of the main issues that men of all age groups. Recent research has revealed that low T and sleep are linked. While low T is often by sleep deprivation, insomnia can result in low testosterone levels. Insufficient sleep can lead to stress and increase cortisol, the stress hormone. The increase in levels of cortisol can cause lower testosterone levels.

Chemicals: They are chemical preservatives, which can be used in products for personal care such as shampoos, conditioners, shaving creams, and lotions. Parabens disrupt the hormone system. When they enter the body through cosmetic products they mimic estrogens and connect to estrogen receptors in your cells. This means that the hormones are released even though they're not intended to release. A higher level of parabens in your body can cause lower testosterone levels.

Mineral and vitamin deficiencies In order to make testosterone your body needs specific vitamins and minerals. Insufficient minerals and vitamins (Vitamin A, C, D and magnesium) within the body plays a crucial role in the development of low testosterone levels.

Magnesium: The absence or deficiency of magnesium levels in the body deprives the endocrine system in the body. It is a crucial mineral needed for the creation of testosterone.

Zinc: Zinc aids your immune system work properly. It also aid enzymes in processing food items and other nutrients that aid in helping to create proteins. Your glands require zinc in order to begin the production of testosterone, insufficient levels of this mineral may result in low testosterone levels.

Vitamin A: Excessive estrogen levels can result in an increase in testosterone production. Incorporating Vitamin A high-quality foods (carrots and fish, as well as Apricots, dark-leafy green vegetables sweet potatoes, and tropical foods) included in the diet will help reduce estrogen levels and boost testosterone production.

Vitamin C: Vitamin C does not just help to boost the anabolic environment that naturally exists within your body, but it also reduces cortisol. If there's less cortisol in the body, it can increase testosterone levels and the reverse is true.

Vitamin D Vitamin D: One of the main reasons this nutrient can boost testosterone production is its presence in Vitamin D receptors in the glass cells that release testosterone. The right quantity of Vitamin D stimulates the production of testosterone within the body and aids men remain fit and healthy.

The risk of SYNTHETIC TESTOSTERONE

Marketing companies of synthetic testosterone boast many benefits , including young energy, strong female erections and massive muscles, but they do not mention the risks that could be that are associated with synthetic testosterone.

A lot of men have been being caught in this trap. The reality is that testosterone synthetic could provide you with some of these, but there are negative consequences that can be related to the treatment. Exogenous testosterone can cause negative side effects that could occur due to normal metabolism as well as increased levels of testosterone in the body. This article will outline the potential risks which are linked to synthetic testosterone.

Prostate Changes

While testosterone synthetically does not direct cause cancer of the prostate, research studies have shown that higher levels of testosterone can increase the chance of developing prostate cancer in those who are from families with an previous history of prostate cancer or who have been diagnosed with prostate cancer prior to. Prostate enlargement may also happen because of synthetic testosterone as well as the development of prostate cancer cells is accelerated through this increase. Men who are older are at risk, and this is the reason it is advised to stay clear of synthetic testosterone. Prostate growth can result in urinary issues.

Obstetrical Problems with Fertility

The production of testosterone occurs within the testes. It is vital to note that the production of sperm largely relies from this process. The body usually stops producing testosterone once it is supplied by an external source of testosterone. This could be the start of fertility issues.

There is a chance that the testes can cause permanent or significant disruption to producing sperms. that can result in a decrease in the number of sperm. Synthetic testosterone is not recommended for those who hope to start an unplanned family as they may be infertile before a certain age.

The side effect could be either permanent or temporary dependent on the amount of testosterone synthesized present within the body. It is therefore considered a major concern for young men as well as any men who still wish to get more kids. Many men opt for this method following the birth of of children they had planned to have. While some men store their fertile sperm in a bank to protect themselves.

Sleep Apnea

It is a sleep disorder when a person who sleeps stops breathing for a short period of time. There are a variety of medical issues that are caused with this condition, which occurs due to synthetic testosterone. Sleep apnea in the past is often aggravated because of the higher testosterone levels. This is in line with recent research results. The most prominent signs of sleep apnea are regular nighttime sleepiness, and frequent awakening.

The Breasts are enlarged

Synthetic testosterone can cause the breasts becoming tender or expanding breasts. This is common among men of older ages. It is possible that the high levels of testosterone produced by the body could be converted into estrogen, and consequently cause you to begin developing feminine characteristics like larger breasts. Estrogen also affects breast tissue, making it swollen. Both women and men can be affected by estrogen, however those with estrogen levels that exceed the normal range may suffer these adverse effects.

Fluid Retention

The majority of men store fluid in the first few months after testosterone therapy and it could lead to serious health issues, such as the congestive heart condition, an increase in high blood pressure as well as the swelling of ankles and legs. People suffering from congestive heart failure are at chance of suffering heart attacks, as well as other serious heart problems due to the retention of fluid.

The increase of Red Blood Cell Concentration (Polycythemia)

The increase in hemoglobin levels and red blood cell count is one of the most significant results of synthetic testosterone, and it is accompanied by some problems. The older men are also more likely to be experiencing the complications that come with an increased amount in red blood cell.

Some of the most noticeable results of an increase in hemoglobin and blood cells levels are peripheral blood clots that form in the veins of strokes, and heart attacks. This issue can be resolved by blood donation, which decreases the quantity of blood red cells, or by reducing testosterone replacement. The increase in red blood cell count results in blood thickening, that eventually causes hypertension.

It is advised for males to go through a set of tests, which includes the PAS test as well as the rectal exam for prostate cancer, and prostate screening prior to when they are able to receive testosterone therapy. It is essential to have the treatment performed by a qualified professional to prevent certain side adverse effects.

Chapter 3: Rise Testosterone By Consuming

More Nutrients

Testosterone and estrogen are two human sexual hormones that are responsible for growth and reproduction for both genders. They symbolize the desire to be sexually attractive bones, strength and energy, feminine / malevolence, protein production the growth of muscles and hair. Testosterone levels can be increased naturally, without spending a fortune on medications or supplements, simply just by returning to the basic.

Fats and fatty acids

There are three kinds of polyunsaturated fatty-acids: Monounsaturated Fatty-Acids and saturated Fatty-Acids. Certain fats aren't harmful, and your body requires fatty acids for the growth of tissues. Research suggests that 20% to 30% fat content of your food is an best amount to boost testosterone.

Brazil nuts, Avocado's Seeds and Olives are low in saturated fatty acids and are great to snack on.

What is the Saturated Fatty Acids? You can substitute your regular cooking oil with Coconut or Argan Oil, and swap out margarine in favor of real butter, or try Blue Cheese. Real butter offers the benefit of Vitamins A K2, E, and D. Coconut Oil adds a twist to your meals!

Does chocolate have to be forbidden? Raw Cacao or its derivative is a great source of fatty acids. It's packed with anti-oxidant properties, and other benefits from being rich in Magnesium along with Zinc vitamins that also aid in testosterone production.

Cholesterol

It's not all cholesterol harmful, as cholesterol can actually aid in testosterone production. The most common food item in diets all over the world is eggs. Egg yolks are loaded with protein and have an ideal ratio of fatty acids to ensure that everything is in order.

Carbohydrates

The body requires Carbohydrates in fact. They provide your body with energy. Pasta, rice, cereals and breads, as well as potatoes are all complex carbohydrates. There is a good chance that certain of them may already have been in your diet. it could be an exchange (brown into white rice or chips to boiling potatoes) is all that's needed.

For instance, you should include moderate amounts of wheat pasta that is of high quality white rice and wheat-based foods in the diet you eat, as as those leafy green vegetables like Kale, Spinach, Watercress, Pak Choi, Greens, Brussels Sprouts, Broccoli and Cauliflower and even pomegranate have all been shown to decrease the effects of estrogen and boost testosterone levels.

PROTEINS

Proteins are composed of amino acids. They are found in red meats and poultry, pork eggs, fish, eggs however, often beef gelatin is not considered. Gelatin is one of the components in connective tissues, bones and organs of animals.

There have been numerous health reports in recent years regarding gelatin as well as various human illnesses, however, beef gelatin is a good source of Proline and Glycine Two amino acids crucial to the way that our bodies and our brains collaborate (neurotransmitters). They nourish neurotransmitters and improve the body's function and this in turn promotes the purpose of the article.

Go to any health food store or supplement store and you'll find an assortment of BCCA products that contain BCCA. BCCA's have rich in Branch Chain Amino Acids (BCAA's) and are present in dairy products as well as in the protein whey. Research has shown that when coupled with resistance training, the effect of the combination is an increase in testosterone levels. Additionally, there is evidence-based research that suggests any diet that has Omega 3 rich; often found in fish can be beneficial. However, it is important to monitor your protein intake, as studies have shown that diets high in protein may actually have the opposite result and decrease testosterone conversion.

Organic food

Chemicals Pesticides as well as hormones are found within foods and can alter the natural balance of testosterone and estrogen within the body. Organic food is available at a low cost by visiting producers directly or at farmers markets. Make sure you clean all food items prior to eating, since even organic food items may be cross-contaminated.

Foods that surprise you

OYSTERS are a great source of Zinc, Magnesium, Amino Acids, and Vitamin D. It's not the most affordable option, but maybe the passion for this food was more than just their aphrodisiac attributes.

BACON is rich in protein, and contains saturated and cholesterol. All of these are known ingredients that boost testosterone. So you're having you've got that Bacon and Egg breakfast you believed you could quit? Go right ahead.

White button mushrooms, because of their anti-estrogenic qualities, together with Yoghurt bananas, Bananas and Peanut butter have been proven to boost the production of testosterone.

RISE TESTOSTERONE through exercises

Have you ever wondered how prisoners have such distinct bodies? Have you noticed that their diet isn't truly optimal, and they don't supplement their diets and do not have the latest equipment for training?

The majority of what they do is in opposition to the standard advice, which is not to consume less than two grams of protein for every kg of weight. don't train more than 3-4 times a week, drink water continuously Take supplements, and try to exercise for more than 45 minutes per day.

Let me explain you need to know about the key. Testosterone. The hormone that produces anabolic effects in the human body, which assists you in rapidly building muscle mass, and boost bone density, and decrease the body fat percentage.

The majority of people who are in prison are in a relatively high state of testosterone (which can cause more aggressive behavior). However, when they enter an environment where violence is a regular occurrence and they must always watch your back, testosterone levels "explode".

It's all about survival. If you're not big enough, take all of you. In this case, we typically find them training prisoners in the courtyard, using basic weights and compound exercises.

I'm not going to suggest you to go to jail in order to boost the levels of testosterone in your body. I'll discuss more on how exercise affects the testosterone levels and production in your body as well as how exercise can assist you to build the lean and muscular physique that you've always wanted.

How does exercise affect the level of testosterone.

Physical activity, as well as excess physical exercise (over-training) can reduce testosterone levels within the body. Exercise directly impacts testosterone production by stimulating pituitary gland. Exercise can slow down the breakdown of testosterone.

The duration the intensity, frequency and duration of exercise determine the amount of testosterone within the body. The amount increases with intensity of activities with short durations while it decreases for those that last longer, particularly those that require resistance training.

Testosterone production is higher amounts when you perform the heavy (which permits you to perform 5-10 repetitions) and with brief rest intervals between sets of 3 to 5.

The most effective exercises to boost testosterone levels

Compound exercises (as sit-downs using Director, bar, or driven Ramah with dumbbells) will result in a higher testosterone production as opposed to isolation exercises (waving and lateral raises etc.).

When you are using the majority part of the muscles you'll get the most level of testosterone. This means you need to exercise big muscles groups (legs back, chest, legs) with heavy weights.

Normally, the levels of testosterone rise by 30 percent in the morning and by 30 percent in the evening. If you're able start training in the morning to maximize this natural increase.

Research has shown that testosterone levels rise after 45-60 minutesafter exercising. After that the levels of cortisol begin to increase (stress hormone that leads to reduction in muscle mass) and testosterone levels decrease. levels.

Therefore, I suggest you not exercise for longer than 45-60 minutes in a single session.

Naturally increasing your testosterone levels by exercising

Sprint

A variety of scientific tests have proven that you can increase your testosterone levels by sprinting. As one study has shown the testosterone levels rose significantly for those who ran many extremely quick (but extremely intense) 6-second sprints . This was as well as testosterone levels that were always higher even after they were completely restored after the workout.

How can you implement the strategy of sprinting to boost testosterone levels? Try doing a few sprints on the treadmill for fitness after you've placed dumbbells on the gymnasium, or walk out to the backyard, or some kind of playground or the town block and perform a few runs on days or weeks when you're not able to taking into consideration learning.

You can do your own sprints using an exercise bike or an elliptical fitness trainer. Try to incorporate things like 5-10 minutes of sprints when doing a exercise routine, the you will not run for more contrast to 15 for minutes, complete recovery after each run (generally three to four times more than the time the speed you actually ran) In addition, running at least once a week to get optimal results.

Lift Heavy Weights

Although you can do large reps with less dumbbells or even smaller representatives and large dumbbells research has proven that it is usually large dumbbells in order to boost testosterone levels.

The entire system, as well as the massive physical exercises like deadlifts, squats and squats. Regular squeezes, as well as Olympic raises are likely to result in 85-95% or more of the 1RM (or one repetition maximum). You have to do 2-3 whole weight training workout routines each week to have very good testosterone-boosting final results.

If you're a beginner or are just beginning to learn about weightlifting, don't let the idea of intense training to make you feel discouraged. You could replicate a number of these physical exercises using equipment for weight lifting until you're sturdy and capable of using the fat barbell for free or perhaps dumbbell variants.

Employer Long-Term Rest Periods

Professionals analyze the results that show extremely brief rest times for testosterone, as well as discovered that longer rest times of around 120 few seconds for different testosterone supplements are generally superior in producing testosterone (although it is still possible to create different hormones in the body like human growth hormone with shorter rest periods).

Thinking about the issues you've seen while working with massive dumbbells is beneficial as the shorter the duration of your recovery the lower your fat percentage you'll lift. It could also seem like a waste of time to start sitting on the weights at 3 minutes intervals throughout each exercise.

If your goals are generally to increase testosterone levels I would suggest that you increase the training time by doing different actions during the long rest periods such as stretching, or possibly exercising in ways that not put pressure on the same muscular tissues you've previously worked.

As an example for instance, if you're able do a substantial set of regular squeezes, rest for less than 30-60 seconds in several seconds then perform a hefty set of squats. Repeat this process until your entire workout is generally done. You'll also have twice as much amount completed in half the time, yet still getting the benefits of testosterone boosting training in a big way, and also extended rest periods.

Make use of pressured distributions

To perform some form of repeated pushed, do an exercise with weights that targets many of your reps as you can. Then, add a companion (a "spotter") to work together while you finish several more repetitions (anywhere between 1-5 reps).

Research suggests that this representative set produces more testosterone than just performing a number of members as you would do by yourself.

It is better to do reps that are pushed, which include an extensive power-plant with multiple joints. move. As an example you can do an exercise to warm up of squats with barbells. After that you can do it with a partner or personal fitness coach or even someone on the gym for assistance select a fat that allows you to do 5-6 reps by yourself however, it requires the partner to complete another three or four reps done, then to complete an overall of 8-10 reps. This can be repeated between 2 and 6 packages.

If you do not have to have pushed representatives on every exercise or set you perform for instance, if you're trying to boost your testosterone levels, it could be particularly beneficial to complete your last set of any exercise in an exercise set that is pushed.

Use Your Feet

In one study that examined the hormone response to weight-lifting, subjects were placed into an arm-only class as well as a leg-plus-arm class. The increase in testosterone was significantly higher in the class that be incorporated into the decrease in system education along with upper body training.

While it could be appealing people to do physical exercises like biceps curls, along with regular pushing, you'll notice more favorable results with regards to lean body weight, vitality, sexual libido, and weight loss if you incorporate things like multi-joint leg exercises, like lunges for example and squats in your personal program.

Prevent Continual Cardio exercise

Long-term endurance sports like cycling, are believed to reduce testosterone, just as exercise and weight lifting may raise the amount of testosterone. As an example an investigation conducted in 2003 found high levels of testosterone were dramatically lower for cyclists in comparison with weightlifters of a similar age as well as those in those who were not properly trained to manage.

Some experts also suggested that this lower testosterone levels in endurance athletes is a result of a change that gives cyclists, or even athletes with a competitive edge. This is because the leaner muscle that results from testosterone might reduce the speed of the speed of a person.

Therefore when you're looking to boost testosterone levels, you should avoid long runs on the treadmill. Also, it is important to be in agreement with the notion that if you're planning to race marathons or do an Ironman triathlon, perhaps you need to compromise on lower levels of testosterone.

Chapter 4: Essential Supplements

It is likely that you have discussed the importance of testosterone to your body several times. You're likely to know that it's an hormone that is essential in maintaining all the "manly" items. One of the main functions testosterone performs is in sex function and reproduction in addition to other important functions that the body performs such as the level of red blood cells as well as overall health and well-being.

This hormone is well-known for its fluctuation when men age because it is linked to decreased testosterone levels as men age. While age is a major element that causes decreased testosterone levels but other elements that are biological or inherited are also a factor in the decrease levels of the hormone that is vital to. The lower levels can be the cause of a decline in sexual drive, muscle mass or hair growth, and other things. These changes might not be anticipated and cause feelings of inadequacy for the male.

It's good to know that that testosterone deficiency can be treated. Due to their negative effects numerous people are seeking to lessen the negative side effects and return to normal functioning. When people think of increasing testosterone levels, they often immediately think of synthetic substances and illicit supplements that have been linked to adverse unwanted side effects.

But, there are also safe and natural methods to boost testosterone levels, which are essential to know if are having lower levels of testosterone.

Let's examine a few of them and provide healthier alternatives.

Vitamins

Vitamins are known to be the essential elements of our body functions. They are mostly supplied by diet and help our bodies perform different functions in order to keep the balance of health. Vitamin deficiencies are believed to be a major cause of hormonal imbalances such as the lower levels of testosterone.

To increase your testosterone levels of testosterone, you must start by eating a healthy diet. Since a healthy diet is the primary protection against deficiency as well as deficiency of essential vitamins, it is essential to improve it in order to help you achieve your objectives to increase testosterone levels.

A healthy and balanced diet is an excellent beginning. It makes sure that your body gets all the nutrients and vitamins it requires. But, focusing on specific vitamins known to boost testosterone levels is another method to maximize the benefits of your workout.

Foods like avocados and eggs, berries, and pomegranates provide you with many important nutrients and vitamins to increase your levels.

In addition, taking vitamins, particularly vitamin D C along with Vitamins B6, B6 and E will ensure that your levels are in balance. These vitamins are crucial in maintaining your body's healthy functions, and helping you get the most benefit from your food.

Deficiencies in Vitamin A are associated with the decrease in testosterone, and the opposite rise in estrogen, which is a female hormone. By increasing the levels of these vitamin A in the body creates the balance that existed prior to the decrease of these vitamins to be restored , and allow your body to naturally increase the production of testosterone.

Selecting the right vitamins will not only help to get your testosterone levels, but they will also aid in other areas. For example, a well-balanced diet that includes the essential vitamins can help the body help maintain and improve the health of your weight and bodily functions. It's also an essential aspect of maintaining an ideal cardiovascular and heart system.

Minerals

Minerals are similar to vitamins, but they differ slightly in their function within the body. Minerals found in nature as well as consumed by the body via food are safe and healthy. They can also aid in returning the hormone levels in equilibrium. Minerals are widely acknowledged to be the cause of the production of anabolic hormones.

Testosterone is anabolic hormone which is why minerals play a role in its production and maintaining healthy levels. In addition, the absence of minerals in the body could result in low testosterone levels.

While minerals provided through food and a balanced diet can be utilized in our bodies, it is possible that they might not be present in sufficient amounts to work effectively to boost amounts of testosterone. In this instance supplementing with mineral supplements is an option to provide your body with the required quantities of minerals.

Minerals like Zinc magnesium, zinc and Calcium are known as contributing factors to good levels of testosterone. Studies and research on Zinc in the body have revealed that when taken in, Zinc supplements increase testosterone levels by up to 40%..

A consistent consumption of these minerals provides the body to get the necessary supplements to aid in the production of testosterone and restore normal levels. The advantages of using minerals go far beyond just completing the job at hand, and this is the primary benefit of taking minerals from nature instead of synthetic ones that can be harmful to your body.

GUIDE TO TESTOSTERONE NUTRITION

This is a nutrition plan that provides your body with plenty of the most powerful hormones in the world to help you develop optimal muscles. Why was I saying the most significant hormone? Although other anabolic hormones such as insulin affect the growth of muscles but we know for certain that testosterone has the highest potent.

It is not just responsible for growth in muscles, it is a plethora of qualities which make it the most significant hormone, including masculine characteristics like powerful muscles as well as deep voice and hair growth. It also keeps you slim by boosting metabolism, and increases the release of fat cells, and also reduces the storage of fat within the body.

A visit to the gym and taking part in early morning workouts can be a great way to increasing your testosterone levels, but there are other strategies to boost the levels. In order to keep your testosterone levels high, out doesn't mean that you need to turn to illicit steroids or prohormones.

Before heading to your nearest store for supplements to boost the amount of testosterone in your body, consider to boost testosterone levels by adjusting the foods you consume. Knowing what you should eat will be a huge difference to keep your testosterone in the right place to build muscle.

Your diet also influences the production of testosterone. Testosterone circulates in the body in the form of active or free testosterone, or as a binder protein. It is active testosterone that can boost the size of muscles through the muscles cells.

In certain tissues, such as brain cells and fat cells fat cells, fat is converted into estrogen, which are female-specific hormones you should not have over-production in your body since it can cause the accumulation of fat and is a factor in testosterone production. Here are a few qualities you must always include within your food.

Calories

To boost the testosterone level, the most important stage is to consume the right amount of calories. The consumption of a diet that is low in calories will result in lower levels of GnRH being released from the brain. It also results in also a reduction in testosterone catalyzing enzymes found in male testes. The consequence of both events is a decrease in testosterone production.

It is also not advisable to eat excessively and gain weight since it is loaded with enzymes that convert testosterone in to estrogen. A balanced diet will provide enough calories to boost testosterone levels and support for muscles without putting on body fat. The average calorie intake should be between 18 and 20 calories per pound of weight.

Carbohydrates

The second major thing to do is to consume enough carbohydrates. Aim for at least 2 grams for every pound of body weight every day, while keeping the ratio of carbs to proteins at 1:1. Studies have shown that this ratio is the ideal way to boost testosterone levels.

Although it is not often recommended to eat less refined food, I recommend doing it in this case since a diet high in fiber reduce testosterone levels. White rice is a good choice over brown rice because brown rice has a high levels of fiber. However, since you require fiber to maintain your health why not add entire bread and vegetables, and fruits in your diet.

Proteins

This should be the first thing you do. Do not miss this opportunity. 3. You might be shocked to discover that this wasn't No.1. The majority of people are constantly preaching about that importance of taking protein however, taking too much in your diet could affect your outcomes. It's equally important however the most crucial factor is making sure you consume just the right amount but not excessively.

Research has shown that eating lots of protein rather and carbohydrates can lower testosterone levels through urine. Therefore, you should consume 1 one gram of protein for every pounds of body weight every day and no more, no less. Be sure that the majority of your protein comes from animal sources and vegetable-based diets, as they are believed can lower testosterone levels, especially for males. Red meat is beneficial because it contains high levels of zinc and saturated fat This mineral is linked with testosterone levels high.

Fats

This is the final, but certainly not the last. It is suggested that you consume about 30 percent of your calories from fats, but be cautious not to overdose on polyunsaturated oils like those found in fish vegetables oils, salmon and other fish that are fatty. Instead, focus on monounsaturated oils like those found in avocados, nuts olives, olives, and unsaturated fats from egg yolks as well as red meat.

Certain oils, such as olive oil could be on the label, indicating testosterone, which could cause some to be concerned about their health. Studies shows that saturated fats found in chicken, pork and beef are not a cause of increased LDL or bad cholesterol levels.

The spread of your fat consumption over the day to aid in avoiding eating high fat meals which lower testosterone levels briefly.

Shakes for Workout

It is a must to include shakes for post-workout and pre-workout. Consumption of fast digesting protein and fast-digesting carbohydrates after exercise has been shown to boost amount of testosterone. You should aim for no less than 20g of protein along with 20 - 40 grams of carbs prior to exercise and 25-45g of protein and 50 - 100 grams of carbohydrates following exercise.

Vegetables

Consume more vegetables such as the cauliflower Brussels sprouts, broccoli and kale, as well as cabbage, collard greens, turnip greens and arugula. of which are rich in phytochemicals which lower estrogens that are harmful and reduce the testosterone's negative effect.

Be aware of your drinking habits. There are some health benefits to alcohol, but excessive consumption reduces testosterone levels through increasing levels of the testosterone hormone into estrogen. Limit your consumption to less than a couple of glasses per week.

This is an example of the daily menu plan that was designed to boost testosterone levels.

Breakfast

4 eggs in total

Avocado

2-slices of Wheat bread

Morning snack

1 banana

Low fat yogurt

Lunch

Avocado

4 oz. turkey

2 slices of whole wheat bread

Snack before working out

2 slices of white bread

1 tablespoon peanut butter 1 tablespoon peanut

Post-workout snack

1 scoop protein in water

Dinner

1 cup white rice (cooked)

1 cup of cauliflower (cooked)

6 oz. sirloin steak

Evening snack

1 oz. mixed nuts

This is merely an illustration of a diet which includes all the components needed to boost testosterone levels. It contains 3000g of calories and 111g of fat. It also has three hundred grams of carbs. When you adhere to the above-mentioned diet, you'll notice the changes.

Chapter 5: Testosterone Training Guide

Testosterone is the most important hormone in steroidal form that is a major factor in the well-being and health of all males. If your testosterone levels are low, this can have a significant impact on all aspects in your daily life and especially on your sexuality. The libido of your partner will decrease and you could quickly get exhausted, and it can be challenging to get and keep an erection and sperm production is less.

Low testosterone levels may also cause the production of body fat depression, mood swings and insomnia. If you are suffering with any one of the above conditions Don't rely on artificial testosterone supplements. These could have negative consequences of their own. Follow our natural seven-day testosterone-boosting guide and you'll soon be feeling like a man once more.

Day One: Legs Work Out

Exercise is beneficial for your body as well as your mind, it's something that everybody knows however, did you know that doing too much exercise or working out over a long period of time at the same time could be detrimental for the levels of testosterone in your body? It's because they trigger an increase in your cortisol levels and result in a decrease in testosterone. These testosterone-boosting exercises are intended to be done in short, intense bursts. They will result in rapid and effective outcomes.

Begin day 1 in the program with your legs. After a quick warm-up begin with ten jump squats that you repeat five times. The next task is to move a weight or kettlebell between your legs for up to eight times for three sets. The rest period is followed by an calf raise. You can rock forwards and backwards with your calves 10 times while lifting weights. Repeat it three times. The last leg workout involves three sets of weight-bearing lunges. The range is between five to ten times for each leg.

Day 2: Rest Day

The time you take to rest after a hard workout is just as essential for the testosterone levels of your body as the exercises themselves. It is important to strike the right equilibrium between building muscle and increasing testosterone, as well as the excess cortisol production that may result from exercising too often. Day two will be your first rest day before we begin working on the chest and shoulder region.

Day Three Day Three: Chest and Shoulder Workout

A muscular and wide chest is commonly thought of as an indication of masculinity which is also an indication of a high testosterone level. The workout for day three of our testosterone-boosting training guide will also help you get your chest and shoulders in excellent shape. Begin with ten bench presses 5 times. Next, you'll need an inclined bench as you'll be performing 4 sets of 10 dumbbell presses in the inclined angle. Then, press dumbbells vertically from an upright position. Once more, do ten repetitions, however this time in three or four sets. This is a workout that is set for the most difficult finale. The next task is to complete ten reps of an lateral raise standing with dumbbells, either two or three times, then followed by a bent-over lateral raise using the same amount of repetitions and sets.

Day Four: Rest Day

You may already feel the effects of your testosterone-boosting exercises, but don't be tempted to go overboard. Quick, sharp, and powerful workouts are the ones that yield the most effective results when you are looking for a natural method to increase testosterone production. It is equally crucial when it comes to taking a break between sets. Take a break for sixty seconds or so between sets, instead of the 3 to 5 minutes.

Day Five The Back and Arms Workout

Day 5 of our testosterone-boosting workout program focuses on your back and arms as the most powerful indicator of the strength that high testosterone levels can provide. Start with ten pull-ups that are repeated five times. Simply lower your body to straighten the back and bend it while you pull on the barbell. Then, you'll be using your body weight as the goal, as you complete four sets of 6 to 10 pull-ups.

Your body determines the amount of weight you will be doing and it's that classic dip exercise. Perform ten dips over four sets, but remember that you need to dip your body completely and then take your arms to allow it for it to count as dips. Biceps curls follow the next step, and you should try to do ten reps in four sets. Complete your workout with an alternate dumbbell curl. You must do 10 of these in succession using each arm at least three or four times.

Day Six: Rest Day

You should by now begin to notice changes in the way you appear and feel. Your energy levels as well as your natural sexual desire will increase because testosterone begins to increase. The sixth day is your last day of rest, so take care not to take this day off for long cycles or long runs which can reduce the testosterone levels. You can boost your testosterone levels throughout your week with plenty of sleep and eating well by following our testosterone-boosting nutritional guide.

Day Seven Day Seven: Full Body Workout

In our week-long testosterone workout plan, you've been working out various areas of your body. However, seven days later, it's time to tackle the entire body workout. Be aware that these exercises were designed for fast and power-based, rather than sporting activities or exercises that require and increase endurance.

Begin by warming up, and begin with bench presses. Eight repetitions spread over four sets. These will be followed shortly by the exact same number of Squat thrusts. Take a step on all fours then pull your legs towards your stomach, and then return to the side again, vertically behind you for each squat.

The next step is eight barbell deadlifts for four sets. These follow by eight sets of pull-ups. Complete your entire body workout by sprinting six times. Do as quickly as possible for 10 seconds, stop for one minute, then repeat for six sets. Do not be afraid to lower the intensity of any of these goals over the course of the week, particularly in the beginning of the process of increasing you testosterone level, just you must be willing to go for it.

These exercises won't take a lot of time, and when you repeat the program every week, our testosterone-boosting training program will make a huge difference in your life.

Chapter 6: Life Style And Behavioral

Modifications

Relaxation time

Stress, no matter if it's due to your personal circumstances, work-related, or the rush-hour traffic is a Testosterone cause of death. This is because stress increases your body's production Cortisol hormone. When the amount of Cortisol rises within the body, it hinders the body's natural process of testosterone.

Relaxation: Do something every now and then. This could include reading, relaxing and contemplating. Learn to stay away from sweating the small things, even though this might require some effort. Other actions you can adopt to manage your stress include:

It's about getting up and taking a walk each when you're feeling overwhelmed.

Training for breathing exercises that require deep breaths.

Try to be resilient anytime you feel exhausted.

- Listen relaxing instrumental music.

Real Sex with more

The levels of testosterone increase each when you go out for a sexual contact. Contrary to what was believed previously testosterone increases men's sexual libido, resulting in an increase in sexual desire, sex actually is the reverse-it results in high testosterone. In the absence of sex, contrary, lowers testosterone levels. Be aware that this is real sexual activity, not masturbation, which offers little or no, psychological or physiological advantages.

Diet

If you consume lots of foods that are high in sugar like sugary foods like candy, bread, soda and even cookies, blood sugar levels increase in your blood. Thisin turn, lowers the testosterone levels of your body a significant quantity. Research has proven that one sugar-rich food can cause testosterone levels to decrease by as much as 25 percent. If this happens repeatedly in a prolonged period, testosterone levels that are low will likely to occur.

Solution: gradually but slowly reduce your intake of sugar-rich foods and shift to foods rich in carbohydrates since they don't cause an spikes in blood sugar levels. Examples of such foods are whole grains, vegetables, and fruits with low sugar levels like apples and berries.

Diet plays a significant factor in your metabolism of testosterone. The body's glands need minerals like Zinc or Magnesium to begin the process of producing testosterone, while Leydig cells require cholesterol to make the identical. A higher intake of cholesterol and fat consequently, leads to more testosterone levels. People who are on low fat diets have lower testosterone levels. This means that for you to keep your testosterone levels low conditions, eating a diet that is rich in fats is necessary.

Sleep

By staying all night, you increase the chance of not only food binge eating, but also slowing down your metabolism. The body needs adequate sleep. Make sleeping your top priority. Studies have shown that males who sleep less than five hours each night suffer from up to 15 percent decline in testosterone levels.

This means that sleeping is as vital as any other thing you do. In reality, the reason young men feel morning wood is due to the fact that our bodies make plenty of testosterone while we are asleep. The total amount of sleep is directly related with the quantity of testosterone in the morning we've got. The more you sleep, the more testosterone-rich you will be. Therefore, for the best testosterone boost, increase your sleeping duration as well as the quality of your sleep.

Have a good time in the sun.

People who have enough vitamin D present in their blood levels have more levels of T as compared to people with smaller levels. The best method to acquire vitamin D is to expose yourself to sunlight for around 15 to 20 minutes. daily.

Vitamin D can be replenished through daily doses. Vitamin D is associated with improved performance in sports. Experts suggest taking vitamin D3 in the form of supplements every day in order to increase your levels to a normal range. To get a more precise dose make sure to consult your physician who is the most qualified to determine the optimal daily dosage.

Keep in shape.

Weight loss is perhaps the most important thing you accomplish to increase your levels of testosterone. When you shed weight, you can reduce the risk of a variety of other diseases. To combat the problem of excess weight, you should eat fewer processed carbohydrates, such as gluten and sugar. Instead, you should eat a lot of fruits and vegetables. Get enough proteins and fats to build muscle.

Testosterone levels have been discovered to be the highest after two days of exercise. Furthermore, the harder you work out, the more the natural levels of T rise. When you train you should do various compound exercises, like benches presses, squats, as and seat rows that incorporate heavy weights . Your T levels will rise dramatically.

Examples of heavy weights are the use of weight bands or resistance band. To begin, you can hire an instructor to show you the correct technique and form. Make sure you sweat during your workout. The goal is to push your heart harder to reach your testosterone goals, while also losing weight.

Cold baths

Bathing in cold water can increase T levels. Many studies have demonstrated that concentrations of Testosterone in males right after taking a cold shower are extremely high. Because cold showers are readily accessible, anyone looking to increase their testosterone levels ought to consider it. It is not just advantageous as far as t levels are concerned. It can be energizing and beneficial in developing discipline that is vital when you exercise.

Chapter 7: What Should I Know To Be Aware Of

Regarding Your Testosterone Level?

The reality is that around age 30 , testosterone levels in men decrease by around one percent each year. And when they reach 40, they fall by approximately 2% each calendar year.

As we grow older well-nourished to mid age and finally, to older men our normal ranges diminish as does the overall health and well-being.

The first step is to check your testosterone levels and check whether you have testosterone levels that are normal.

Kits for saliva testing at home are available to make saliva testing more convenient.

The test kits that I have used from Opti Male company online, can be found at http://www.checkmytestosterone.com.

The doctor may also conduct and cost-effective blood draws and provide the same results for testosterone levels in total and guidelines for treatment with hormones should you be a suitable candidate.

Monitoring your testosterone levels and making sure you check them regularly is the most effective method to monitor your progress and stay on your best level.

Testing for nutrition is another great method to detect micronutrient and vitamin deficiency.

A company such as SpectraCell offers testing clinics throughout the world. You can go to http://www.spectracell.com and look under find a clinic, that does micronutrient testing for vitamins, minerals, amino acids and antioxidants or your doctor may be able to perform these tests as well.

Important to Maintain Testosterone Levels

Many men experience the negative effects of low testosterone every day and the majority live throughout their lives unaware that it can be managed by supplementation, diet, exercises, and sometimes the use of hormone therapy.

Low testosterone levels are accompanied by an array of signs which can seriously impact men's health overall, typically beginning with weight gain, stomach fat, mood swings as well as a decrease in libido and the loss of muscle mass.

The majority of men view testosterone as a hormone for muscle. Testosterone does not only control muscle but also regulates the body's fat. Insufficient testosterone levels can cause an increase in belly fat and stomach fat.

The excess body fat that results from low testosterone can be very hard on the arteries, and could result in decreased blood flow.

Low T may also cause damage to brain cells and neurons that can affect not only the way we feel and appear but also impact the way we think.

Where do I begin?

It's a common belief that obesity , poor diets, fast food, and other unhealthy practices can cause low testosterone levels.

If after testing you are in the normal to below the average, then taking the normal route is what I and a lot of individuals have attempted to keep and even increase our T levels to levels that are higher than what the majority of men of our age will ever be able to.

Start with diet, exercises and a few simple lifestyle adjustments, you can significantly reduce the severity of ailments that are associated with low T.

The process of optimizing your T levels using the testosterone-boosting blueprint can be a huge impact and we'd like to show you how to achieve this and help you get back to looking and feeling great once more.

Whatever your health, age or situation the program is suitable for anyone who is willing to make some changes in his lifestyle and commit an insignificant period of time.

What are the most effective diets to shed excess weight, build muscles and increase T levels?

The Optimal Caloric Intake

We discussed earlier the importance of diet and optimal caloric intake as the main ingredient in this program.

It is the first thing to do. determine what you are getting in your caloric consumption each day.

How many calories per everyday basis are you taking in?

It is possible to track your calories over a couple of days and then compute an average. To get more precise, you could use a nutritional food scale such as the Escali brand, which monitors sodium, calories proteins, fats carbs, and even fiber. Or, you can look up the chart of calories for totals on the packaging of foods you're taking in.

Most men should fall in one of three categories.

1: If you're looking to lose 20lbs or more and increase your muscle mass. Multiply the weight of your body times 11.

Example: 210 pound man. 210 x 11 = 2310 total calories per day.

2310 calories is the daily caloric requirement until you have reached your goal.

2. If you're looking to lose some weight around your middle, and also build muscles. Multiply your body weight times 15.

Example: 190 pound man. 190 x 15 = 2850 total calories per day.

2850 calories is your daily caloric intake until you have reached your goal.

3. If you're thin and looking to build muscles. Multiply your body weight times 19.

Example: 170 pound man. 170x19 = 3230 total calories per day.

Important Notes

If you're currently eating more than your ideal amount of calories, begin to reduce your intake slowly over the period of one couple of weeks rather than all at one time.

If you're looking to increase your the weight of your muscles, slowly begin adding calories over several weeks until your body is adjusted.

If you are in a highly busy job, you might want to add a few extra calories to your goal.

If you're looking to change your diet and shed weight before beginning an exercise program, it's okay.

The sooner you integrate exercise into your diet, the more effective and quicker the outcomes.

Making realistic goals, creating new habits, and progressing in time will alter your body shape, shed or gain weight, and increase testosterone levels.

Optimal Nutrient Intake

Making sure you are getting the proper quantities of the three micronutrients is crucial.

The three micronutrients that are important to us are carbohydrates, proteins and fat.

It is your goal to keep a balance these three factors at each food intake, and also to meet your daily caloric goal.

In the subsequent chapters, we will present an eating plan for weight loss, as well as a diet plan to build muscle.

Proteins

Proteins are the basic building blocks of life. They build and repair body tissue, cartridges bone and organs, as well as connective tissue.

The recommended daily dose for males that exercise frequently is around 1 grams of protein per kilogram of bodyweight.

Even though consuming the proper amount of protein is important but you shouldn't consume more protein than carbohydrates as it may decrease your testosterone levels.

Proteins aren't just important in developing muscle as well as increasing the T level it's also a great fat burnersince your body is required to take longer to digest proteins than carbohydrates. Proteins require about 2 hours to absorb.

81

Consuming up to 30 grams of protein after awakening can boost how you feel and aid in helping you shed weight.

Proteins made from whey are an excellent source of protein, and they are absorbed faster within the human body.

Proteins from Casein are taken in slowly and are effective while whey proteins remain a great source of protein they are taken in more rapidly in the human body.

Incorporating your daily protein needs with protein shakes and bars during meals is the best way to make sure you hit your desired protein levels each day.

Carbohydrates

If you're looking to shed just a few pounds, or 20 pounds or more within the shortest period of time feasible, eating slow-digesting carbohydrates is the best way to move.

The first step towards losing weight is to avoid all starchy or white carbohydrates like white bread pasta, rice as well as cereals, potatoes and other grains.

All of these are high-glycemic foods that could raise the blood sugar levels of your body.

Beware of simple sugars such as fruit juices and fruits.

Avoid trans fats like margarine, processed food products and oils such as corn, soy and safflower.

The most effective examples of slow-digesting carbs and low-glycemic food are leafy green vegetables such as broccoli, spinach as well as asparagus, cauliflower whole wheat breads and pastas.

Legumes and beans are also a excellent source of protein, such as pinto beans, black beans red beans, soybeans and black beans.

By switching your carbohydrate consumption to a low-carbohydrate diet, and avoiding white carbs even without exercising, the majority of men can shed up to 20 pounds within 30 days or less.

Take a look at our slow carbohydrate mix-and match meal plan from the next chapter. Pick some meals you could repeat until you achieve your weight loss goals.

One of the greatest benefits is that you can eat whatever you want throughout the day, and even have a cheat day every week, where you can eat whatever you want and even junk food.

The Fat Consumption (eating fat does not cause you to be fat)

The amount of fat you consume will comprise between 20 and 30% of your daily diet and is one of the most essential elements in maintaining and increasing you testosterone levels.

Testosterone, along with other essential male hormones are made by cholesterol, a healthy fat that the body produces by digesting fats. If you are deficient in your body, testosterone levels will drop.

The most important thing is to eat healthy fats that are healthy for us.

The best fats are monounsaturated, polyunsaturated as well as saturated.

Monounsaturated fats can be found within avocados, canola oils and nuts such as almonds that are raw pecans, cashews, pecans as well as Brazil nuts.

They can also be found in olives, olive oil almond butter, peanut butter, sunflower oil, and dark chocolate.

The polyunsaturated fats can be found in corn oil. fat fish in cold water such as mackerel, herring and salmon as well as tuna, sardines and trout.

They are also present in flax seeds and pumpkin seeds, as well as sesame seeds and sunflower seeds.

The saturated fats can be found in animal sources such as red meat as well as poultry and dairy products.

Consuming a variety of whole eggs every day are excellent sources of saturated fats and cholesterol. They give you the essential fatty acids that are essential for maintaining healthy hormone levels.

All of these boost testosterone levels, decrease bad cholesterol, decrease the risk of heart disease, and stabilize blood sugar levels and even fight against certain types of cancer.

If possible, consume higher-quality meats and fruits and vegetables, like grass fed beef, organic vegetables and fruits.

When and for how long? times in a day are we supposed to consume?

As you can notice in our menu plans, you'll be eating multiple times per day, breaking down the calories into small meals.

A regular diet will provide an ongoing intake of nutrients, and also forces your body to create more testosterone. It is possible to eat at least four meals per day, and three to four meals between meals.

The most important breakfast of the day is breakfast and you shouldn't skip breakfast!

After a night of sleep, your body is dehydrated, nutrient deficient state the moment you awake.

Drinking plenty of water and eating proteins within the first 30 mins of getting up is a good way to establish and you can enjoy your main meal shortly afterwards.

In between meals, having snacks daily is a good habit to establish.

My favorite protein bars are protein shakes along with assorted nuts and dried fruits.

Mix of slow-burning carbs and match Meal Plan

Men who want to shed weight The chart below can be a great mixing and matching, eating everything you like in your food items.

In the next 30 days and in conjunction with exercising, select three or four combinations of meals from the menu below, and repeat, and then enjoy.

Cheat Day

You can have a cheat day during this diet. This means that every week, on on a weekend or a day when you are allowed to eat anything you like, everything!

It's true that this cheat day can boost your body's metabolism and help you increase and burn fat.

Mix and match food lists

Egg whites 1 to 2 whole eggs

Thigh or breast of chicken

Fish

Pork

Beef

Legumes

Lentils

Black beans

Soybeans

Red beans

Pinto beans

Vegetables

Mixed Mixture - cauliflower/broccoli

Peas

Asparagus

Spinach

Broccoli

Sauerkraut

Green beans

Important Tips

You'll be losing electrolytes and water on this diet. Drink lots of fluids and avoid dairy, soy milk soft drinks, or juices from fruit. 2 glasses of red wine is acceptable.

Avoid all white carbs Bread, rice, and bread (even brown) pasta, cereals tortillas, and fried foods.

If you're eating out in a dining establishment, switch your rice with vegetables.

Muscle Mass and Gain Meal Plan

Here's a sample four-week menu plan that will provide your body the right proportion of protein, calories and fats to increase your testosterone levels.

This sample is of the lean weight of a 200 pound man who is looking to build muscular mass.

The meals we recommend on our menu plans can increase your testosterone levels and help you build endurance and stamina.

The more effort you devote to your workout routine and daily routine, the more energy you'll receive back.

What are the most effective testosterone-boosting supplements?

I've personally tried and tried many T boost supplements available that are available Some of them have been removed from the market. For good reason. They could cause harm for your health.

I've got a small checklist of products that proven to work extremely well for me. I am finding myself repeating them time.

Be aware when you take supplements. Using untested multi-vitamins that make large promises of higher testosterone levels and building muscle can be risky and very hard on your kidneys and liver.

Take supplements only in the manner recommended by your doctor or consult your physician if you have any concerns or questions.

Selling and marketing of supplements that are not regulated is a major business and the only ones who profit are the companies that make them. They employ the " keep consumers confused to make a profit".

The following supplements are the ones I depend on frequently and which has been proven by numerous studies to be the most effective all-around supplements for resistance training. I exercise weights three to four times a week.

L-glutamine

Helps reduce suboptimal food absorption. Supplements and foods are useless unless they are properly absorbed.

It can also speed up the healing process and prevent soreness after exercise.

It is possible to load L-glutamine during the first 5 days and use it as a post-workout supplement.

The amount of food you consume: up to 80 grams daily 10 grams every couple of hours.

Maintenance: 10-30 grams after workouts (powder is the best)

Creatine Monohydrate

Increases force production and protein production. Enhances strength size, power and strength. Enhances the levels of specific important anabolic hormones.

Safe level: 5 - 20 grams daily.

Training days 10-grams 30 minutes prior to the workout.

Days off from training: 5 grams at the time of waking and 5 grams prior the bed.

Cissus Quadrangularis

Reduces the accumulation of fat and reduce cortisol levels, which could lead to an increase in testosterone and the development of new muscles tissue.

Helps rebuild joints, muscles ligaments, bone and joints.

Consume 1600 mg during meals and breakfast.

Alpha Lipoic Acid

A antioxidant that has glucose elimination capabilities that result in greater weight loss as well as insulin-sensitive.

300 mg taken 2 - three times per day 30 minutes before all-food meals.

Branch Chain Amino Acids

Aids in promoting hormone production. reduce fatigue and muscle breakdown and

Improves nitrogen retention for restore and repair muscles.

Eat between meals, 30 minutes prior to workouts, immediately following workouts.

Zinc

Aids in promoting the repair of tissues, muscle growth as well as testosterone production.

Take 50mg once a day in conjunction with meals.

Daily Supplements

Good multivitamin that is 100 percent RDA of C, E as well as magnesium, calcium along with vitamin D.

Omega-3 fish oil omega 3 fats, EPA and DHA.

EPA is a good source of oxygen within the body.

DHA is vital in the transmission of signals to the eyes, brain as well as the nervous system.

3000 mg a day - best taken in conjunction with meals.

Testosterone Maintenance:

The oil of cod's liver fermented as well as butter fat (capsules)

To maintain long-term testosterone levels and general wellbeing I make use of Green Pastures blend every day.

You can find this supplement at http://www.greenpastures.com

It is possible to replace this supplement with simple tablet of cod liver oil as well as the use of a high quality butter made from genuine butter fat. Kerrygold Irish Butter is a good choice and can be purchased at the local grocery stores.

Vitamin D-3

Check for Vitamin D3 deficiencies prior to supplementing. At home tests are available online at ZTR laboratories http://www.zrtlab.com

The normal blood level should be 55ng/ml.

3000 IU in the morning and before the bed.

Quick T Accelerating Formula to Improve Sex

Ribeye steak for dinner the night before having sex.

4 eggs of a large size within only a few hours from getting ready for bed the night before.

Brazil nuts, raw almonds and Brazil - consume 3 to 4 Brazil nuts, and 20 or so almonds raw a couple of hours before sex.

Capsules of cod liver oil fermented 2 capsules, 4 hours prior to sexual activity.

What small lifestyle changes can be made to increase T levels?

Be active.

Consumption of Water

The body is 80 percent water, and all of body functions are depended on. The majority of men are in constant dehydration and drink too much tea, coffee soft drinks, alcohol and soft drinks.

Your body requires at least 1 ounce of clean, pure water that is filtered per pound of total body weight each day.

A person who weighs 200 pounds must consume about 100 ounces of water per day.

Drinking water with a clean filter will increase testosterone levels and help keep you healthy.

Many municipal water sources are contaminated with drugs and other substances leftover from human consumption, which could directly affect hormone levels.

Utilize a water filtration pot or choose one which connects to the faucet to make it easier to use.

If you consume bottled water ensure that the bottles that you drink from are BPA non-toxic plastics. The BPA is a chemical that can be absorbed into your water and reduce the levels of testosterone.

Sleeping

The goal is to more restful, better quality sleep and more rest.

The body repairs and renew its self during sleep, and that's the time it starts to activate the T-producing mechanisms.

The more sleep you have, the higher levels of T you'll be able to maintain since HGH is released during sleep phases.

Create a routine of having regular bed and wake times at all times, even on weekends. Also, don't go to bed overstuffed by food or thirsty.

Soaps and Lotions

Check your labels for additives and parabens that may influence your body's normal hormones.

Check labels for words such as butyl, Ethyl and propyls. Avoid them.

Avoid tea and lavender tree oils as they can cause hormonal imbalances between testosterone and estrogen.

Stay Cool

Cold can stimulate fat burning and releases of fatty acids within your body.

Try these simple tips to boost fat-burning.

Take a bath or shower for around 10-minutes at a stretch.

Begin by taking an ordinary shower, then cleanse and then rinse. Gradually reduce the amount of hot water you use until your body is accustomed to cold water.

It's very tough, but also refreshing.

Ice packs offer a smaller version that has similar effects.

Pack ice cubes or ice onto the neck's back and your upper traps for 20-30 minutes, seven days a week.

Cell Phones

Don't carry your cellphone in the front pocket of your purse near to your testicles.

Radiofrequency magnetic radiation may decrease the percentage of mobile sperm, affecting semen quality , and affect male fertility.

What are the top training and exercises to increase your T?

I was once an avid gym-goer, and would spend many hours a week exercising.

Nowadays, I'm more the gym rabbit. I'm out and in as fast as I can, and only rarely do I train for longer than 45 minutes every 3-4 days of the week, at minimum.

Testosterone boosting blueprint has been designed as a minimal program that will give you the best results in the shortest duration.

Exercise and gym time is not any more or less the same. The workout that boosts testosterone requires a five minute warm-up on the treadmill .

Then, 10 minutes or less of multi-joint lifting exercises for the entire body which stimulate the largest muscles and trigger more powerful hormone release.

Each workout should last for shorter than 45 minutes, and you'll only be doing 8 repetitions for each exercise . You should allow 3 minutes of rest between each workout.

This regimen isn't in line with the majority of gym's standard procedures and what the majority of men do, however you can increase strength and size of muscles by not working out as much, eating well and taking more rest!

The most important thing is that every exercise is slowed to a four second increment and a 4 second down instead of the standard 2 seconds upand 2 seconds down.

By counting 4/4, you'll be pressing your muscles to complete failure on the 8th or last rep. The first 7 reps will serve as an exercise to warm up for the 8th repetition.

You will get more muscle time during contraction this way , and using the maximum weight that you can this way, you can do more in less time!

It is only 70% of the max lifting weight, which you can do five times for each exercise. When you are stronger, you'll only add 10 pounds or 10 percent.

We suggest that you work toward completing at least 10 exercises in a workout. However, you can perform 3-5 to begin. Refer to our exercise chart.

I've noticed that as we get older, muscle tissue is slower to recover and the time to recover is more crucial than ever before.

This workout lets you take up to three days of rest between workouts when you are more fit.

To get the best testosterone levels I am of the opinion that resistance training and weight lifting is the best way to go.

The goal of this program isn't to turn you into the next professional athlete or super strong person, but you'll become leaner and stronger after this workout.

Burning Calories

I've seen so many men in the gymand ride stationary bikes, running on treadmills or the steppers on stairs for 30 to 60 minutes at an time. It is true that no exercise can burn off a lot of calories.

If you take one cookie, it's about 100 calories. It would take the treadmill for about an hour to burn off 100 calories.

The most effective way to reduce calories and fat is to build and sustain the muscle mass and increase testosterone levels with the use of weights and resistance.

Training with weights is always the best and will provide the highest quality results in the shortest period of time.

Weight Training

Many people who train tend to overtrain. Training too much can strain your immune system, and increase the chances of getting injured or getting sick.

If you are pushing yourself too hard to burn more fat and calories can stop your body from obtaining the testosterone field it needs.

The exercises that follow will increase your body's T-levels without training too much.

Chapter 8: Essentials For Low Testosterone

Levels As Well As Testosterone Replacement

Therapy

What exactly is Testosterone?

Testosterone is one type of hormone that is produced by the testicles . It is responsible in the proper development of sexual traits in males. Testosterone is also vital for maintaining optimal sexual functions, a feeling of wellbeing, bone growth as well as adequate quantities of blood red cells and maintaining muscle mass.

Insufficient testosterone production isn't an usual cause of Erectile dysfunction can occur because diminished testosterone production. To address the issue it is possible that testosterone replacement therapy can aid.

What causes low levels of Testosterone?

Factors that contribute for the formation of testosterone deficiency are the following:

* Excessive stress that strains the adrenal system.

* Infections such as AIDS that weaken the immune system.

* Inflammatory conditions such as Sarcoidosis (a condition that causes an injury or infection of the testicles)

* Hypogonadism, which is when the test is the inability to produce sufficient levels of testosterone. Also often referred to as androgen deficiency

* Hemachromatosis (excessive levels of iron in the blood)

• Pituitary gland malfunction (the pituitary gland, a gland in the brain, which synthesizes substances that regulate the release of hormones from your brain and into your testis)

* Chronic illness

* Chemotherapy or radiation treatment for cancer that damages or affects the testicles

* Alcoholism

* Some types of medicines especially those employed to treat depression and other mental disorders.

The reason for testosterone levels to decline is unclear and poorly comprehended.

Sublime Symptoms of Low Testosterone

The symptoms and signs of low testosterone are usually obvious, but they may appear subdued. The testosterone levels naturally decline when men age and symptoms may show up gradually. The signs associated with low levels of testosterone are:

• Low feeling of wellbeing

* Irritability

* Depression

* Difficulty in concentrating

Poor energy levels and fatigue

* Erectile dysfunction

* Low libido, or sex drive

If a specific male exhibits signs of low levels of testosterone, and tests show that he does indeed have an insufficient amount of testosterone A doctor may suggest treatments. For the hundreds of males who have low levels testosterone but do not show any symptoms there is no treatment currently recommended.

What changes to the levels of testosterone as you get older?

The levels of testosterone are highest at the time of puberty, and then in early adulthood. As you get older, your testosterone levels slowly fall down - typically around 1 percent per year after reaching the age of thirty. It is essential to determine the reason for this decline in levels of testosterone occur caused by the decline in testosterone due to aging normal or if they are caused by a medical disorder known as hypogonadism.

Do naturally declining levels of testosterone lead to the symptoms and signs of the aging process?

It's not really. Males may experience a wide range of symptoms and signs as they age. Many of them are an effect of low testosterone levels and may include the following:

* Changes in your mood Low levels of testosterone can lead to a decline in confidence and motivation. You might feel sad or sad or have difficulties focusing or remembering things.

* Physical alteration There is a huge possibility of different physical changes like decreased bone density, less strength and bulk, as well as increased body fat. Swollen or tender breasts

(gynecomastia) and body hair loss are likely to happen. You might feel less energetic than you did previously and feel hot flushes.

Changes in your sleep patterns . Often low testosterone levels could cause insomnia and other sleep disorders.

• Changes to sexual functioning which could mean less spontaneous erections like at night, infertility, and decreased sexual desire.

It is important to remember it is possible that these signs are normal occurrences of aging. Other symptoms and signs could result from different conditions, such as the excessive alcohol consumption or drugs, depression, thyroid issues as well as medication-related negative consequences. The only way to detect low testosterone levels is to test for testosterone in blood.

What changes occur in the body due to low levels of Testosterone?

A low level of testosterone may cause the physical changes that follow:

* Changes in the levels of lipids and cholesterol levels

* A decrease in body hair

* Osteoporosis, or bones that are fragile.

* A decrease in hemoglobin levels and perhaps mild anemia

* The levels of cholesterol

* Reduced the mass of muscles, accompanied by the increase of body fat

How can low levels of Testosterone In Men Detected?

The only way for a person to recognize the disease is to see a doctor to take a look at the testosterone levels present that are present in the blood. Because testosterone levels are likely to fluctuate throughout the day, a variety of tests will need to be taken to determine any deficiencies. Doctors would prefer, if they can to test levels of testosterone earlier in the morning since this is the time when testosterone levels are at their highest.

What exactly is Testosterone Replacement Therapy (TRT)

If you discover that you suffer from testosterone levels that are low There are options to your issue. Testosterone Replacement Therapy or TRT is a treatment for males who aren't producing sufficient levels of testosterone. TRT is generally long-term in nature and should only be started after testosterone deficiency has been confirmed clinically, which includes measuring the hormone levels in the lab and removing any other possible health problems.

Testosterone Replacement Therapy is available in a variety of types. Any of them can increase testosterone levels.

The injections as well as Implants - testosterone could be implanted in the form pellets within the soft tissues, or directly injected into muscles. The body gradually absorbs testosterone into the bloodstream.

* Mouth Patch * Mouth Patch Striant is a pill that sticks to the upper gums close to the upper incisor. Testosterone mouth patches are placed every day and they continually releases the hormone into bloodstream via the tissues within the mouth.

* Gels * Gels Testim as well as AndroGel are available as packets of testosterone gels that are clear. If it is applied each day, testosterone gets

directly absorbed by your skin. Fortesta, Axiron and AndroGel are among the most popular testosterone gels that are sold in pumps that provide the amount of testosterone prescribed by a doctor. Natesto is another type of testosterone gel, which is applied through the nose.

*Transdermal (Skin Patch) - an illustration of a commercial version of testosterone skin patches is Androderm that is applied to the upper part of the body or on the arm. Testosterone skin patches can be applied every day.

You may be asking yourself what the point is of taking one testosterone pill? Oral testosterone is readily available but there are health experts who believe that oral testosterone can cause adverse reactions to the liver. Other strategies, like injections, orally tablet disintegration, gels, and patches on the skin, bypasses liver and directly releases testosterone into the bloodstream.

Each one of these options provides enough testosterone, though they all have different advantages and drawbacks. Talk to your doctor to determine which of these options is most appropriate for you.

What exactly is Androstenedione?

It is being advertised commercially as a method to "naturally" increase the levels in testosterone levels, androstenedione actually is an ingredient that is like steroids, which is a metabolite from DHEA and is a natural precursor of testosterone. Androstenedione is generally regarded as a steroidal supplement for dietary intake to control the testosterone levels. If consumed in large quantities it can cause results that are like powerful anabolic steroids, such as testosterone.

Although it can also serve to boost the production of androgens, it should not be regarded as substitute for medical treatments, or as a supplement since it is not yet received approval from the Food and Drug Administration. Companies that sell this type of steroids typically make statements which are false and little is known about potential adverse effects on our bodies of some of these substances. If you require testosterone supplementation, follow the suggestions, treatments and medicines that are prescribed by your doctor.

Who should not take Treatment for Testosterone Replacement Therapy?

Due to the growing use of supplements to boost testosterone and the human growth hormone (HGH) online and in the marketplace, the use of synthetic testosterone is gaining popularity. Its stated purposes are treating infertility, treating problems with sexual drive and low-sex, treating the issue of erectile dysfunction, improving athletic performance , and giving an increase in energy levels. However, TRT can have negative consequences if it is not used correctly as well as, like HGH supplementation, it's not recommended for the most healthy males.

TRT might not be suitable for men who are at risk of developing prostate cancer. Also, it is not appropriate for those with the disease of heart, prostate cancer, or excessive cholesterol levels. The exposure to testosterone has been recognized to trigger certain types of cancerous cells within the prostate glands of vulnerable individuals. Therefore, it is essential for men who are contemplating TRT for prostate cancer to go through a complete prostate cancer test prior to starting the process of TRT.

Does TRT have any side effects?

If the amount of testosterone you receive is sufficient there are negative side consequences. TRT is still not examined thoroughly and the jury isn't yet out about its potential adverse consequences. The most frequent negative side consequences of TRT are:

* Inflammation of the ankles

* Possible liver damage

* The mood swings

A noticeable increase in appetite

* Headaches

* Acne

* Erections or a priapism that doesn't seem to disappear, and can last for more than 4 hours. The condition referred to as Priapism requires immediate medical attention.

* Nausea and vomiting

A few Therapeutic indications for Testosterone Replacement Therapy

Testosterone replacement plays a significant role in treating hypogonadism and can help improve health-related conditions that are related to it, such as Anemia and fatigue. Furthermore many

111

other beneficial effects associated with testosterone supplements have led to a growing interest in its possible applications in the following situations:

* Heart failure with chronic
* Diabetes mellitus
* Diabetes mellitus
* Osteoporosis
* Erectile dysfunction
* Dementia. The research base is not extensive and the balance of benefits must be clarified

A Brief History of Testosterone Replacement Therapy

Organotheraphy, also known as the practice of treating like-to-like it has been practiced for many thousands of years. In theory testosterone replacement therapy also known as TRT is a continuation of the organotheraphy principle. The scientific basis for TRT was created by 3 important pieces of research.

The initial research was carried out during the year 1849 by an zoo's curator from Goettingen,

Germany, named Arnold Berthauld. Berthauld discovered that when the roosters were castrated, they stop from mating, to cuddle or fight. Furthermore the roosters' combings can regress. The normal development of their combs and behaviour can be restored through the transplanting the testes. Then, Berhauld came to the concluding that testes' hormones react on the blood and the blood reacts upon the whole body. This is why the first time that testosterone hormone was discovered and, in actual that is how endocrinology came into existence.

The second research is thought of by many to be among the best instances of self-experimentation within the medical field. In 1889, Charles Edouard Brown-Sequard, who was a 72-year old French physiologist/physician rose before the Society de Biologie of Paris. He declared that he had rejuvenated himself with injections of testicular fluids derived from guinea pigs and dogs.

Therefore, the testicular extract of Brown-Sequard was reported to be completely devoid of androgen hormones. This is despite its benefits are attributed to undoubtedly a result of a placebo. But the concept behind Brown-Sequard's research has resulted in an enormous public interest in the possibilities for testosterone supplements. The growing public and scientific interest generated by the Brown-Sequard research has resulted in the Nobel-winning production of testosterone in the late 1930s and the fact that the medical treatment of hormone replacement therapies (TRT).

In 1944, the last piece of scientific research which defined TRT took place exactly 10 years after the initial success in synthesizing testosterone. In a paper titled "The Male Cliacteric", Gordon Myers and Carl Heller, who are both internists, wrote that some men with age show symptoms that could be explained by hypogonadism.

Insufficient sexual energy, easy fatigability, depression, and memory impairment are a few of the most frequent symptoms. Because the measurement of serum testosterone was not feasible at the moment, Myers and Heller came to the conclusion that it was male climacteric through bioassays and testicular biopsies that indicated higher quantities of urinary gonadotropin. Gonadotropin levels were elevated in castrated and male climacteric and the normal levels of gonadotropins was found in those suffering from psychological impotence and normal men. Myers and Heller added that in men who have high climacteric levels, the levels of gonadrotropin and symptoms returned to normal after the administration of testosterone propionate. The findings of later research have shown that women who have had their ovaries removed as well as suffering from declines in sexual function have seen benefits from taking testosterone. Therefore, testosterone replacement therapy has been beneficial for both genders.

In the past, introducing testosterone to the human body had its own challenges. Initial oral testosterone tablets have caused liver toxicity and remain a problem to make today. The testosterone that can be implanted that is injected under the skin was successful and is still used in the present, but this procedure requires minor surgical procedures that could pose certain risks, such as irritation and infection at the site of implantation. The most commonly used method of testosterone replacement therapy is injections, however modern technologies have led to development of testosterone patches that are less as invasive as testosterone injections.

The benefits from Testosterone Replacement Therapy

The main goal in testosterone replacement therapy isn't to make men happier on a only a superficial scale. It's a shame that this is the opinion of the majority of people. Instead, addressing low levels of testosterone is an essential factor for the preventative and treatment of certain chronic illnesses.

But, improving the quality of life of a man should not be ignored. The procedure in testosterone replacement therapy meant to address emotional, sexual and physical consequences of low testosterone levels.

1. Muscles with a higher elevation Tone and Strength

One of the most frustrating experiences that a man can experience is when you attempt to improve your health overall however your body seems determined to stop any kind of improvement.

That's precisely what happens when testosterone levels decrease.

Whatever you do to strive to maintain your body active the muscles will not be able to maintain their strength and strength.

It is a dangerous practice for men who are older. TRT can help you gain back the toned, strong muscles you used be able to enjoy when you were only 20 years old. A recent study revealed that men who had undergone TRT for just a few months showed an increase in the muscle mass by about 2 and a half pounds.

Don't let a lack of testosterone levels stop you from feeling like an alpha male. The low testosterone level is common for older males. By simply taking TRT you'll notice an immense improvement in the strength of your muscles and strength. In turn, you'll begin to notice remarkable improvements in overall health and wellbeing.

2. More endurance, stamina and Energy

The use of hormone replacement therapy has a huge effects on our general health.

Apart from reducing the likelihood of serious health issues Supplementation with testosterone may be beneficial in addressing even the smallest things, like energy restoration.

In this days and times, every one of us could benefit of a method that can improve our energy levels increase our endurance, and increase our endurance. Testosterone plays an essential role in keeping endurance, stamina and energy levels in balance.

• Benefits to the body

A low level of testosterone may cause an inactive lifestyle. If your body isn't getting the proper amount of exercise that is required it could be afflicted with many issues. Through TRT you is at its optimal level of flexibility and the size of your muscles. This allows your body perform at its peak. A healthy lifestyle that is active into your later years can reduce the chance of developing other ailments and improve your longevity.

Benefits to your Social Life

You may not have realized how your energy levels have gotten until you get back to the testosterone level. In a flash you'll have the energy needed to get out or engage in other things. You will not feel tired even after one flight of stairs, or to keep watching your favourite late-night television shows. The older men tend to lead sedentary lives and the majority of them won't be able to spend moments with loved ones as often as they'd like. Don't let this occur to you.

* Benefits for your personal life

A boost in your testosterone levels improves your endurance and willpower to complete the small tasks you'd like accomplish. Fishing and gardening may not be a chore that is difficult however the testosterone levels of your body aren't high enough for you, you may not be able to sit in the garden even for one hour. A healthy testosterone level can allow you to perform what you'd like to do with no restrictions.

* Benefits to your mental capacity

When you've restored the testosterone levels in the body, you'll be capable of seeing a project through to its completion. This is due to the fact that you be able to focus.

In addition to being competent enough to finish a project but you'll also be more positive about the world around you. Low testosterone levels can lead to anxiety and depression. After the recovery of your hormones, it is possible to be more optimistic about your day-to-day routine. Small issues and setbacks won't be a hassle for you as they were in the past.

The increased stamina is evident in your emotional, mental and physical levels. You'll be able to overcome fatigue, stress and illnesses. The treatment for testosterone replacement will not only help you get back to "normal" but it can also help you feel youthful and energetic. With testosterone levels that are healthy you will be able to live living life to the highest level.

3. Enhanced Memory, Focus and Concentration

In addition to improving your physical well-being, testosterone replacement therapy can also have a significant impact on your mental health. A better mental state leads in improved overall health. Aging may play major roles in the decline in cognitive capacity but it is possible that the ageing process might not be the only factor that is responsible. A low level of testosterone can result in memory loss, difficulty focus and a lack of concentration.

A healthy level of testosterone has been found to improve math-related cognitive abilities of males aged between 35 and 90 years old. By using testosterone replacement therapy you can restore your mind back to a normal or even higher functioning level.

* Concentration

Before beginning the testosterone-replacement therapy could have had lower levels of concentration. Restoring healthy amounts of testosterone will help you regain the focus you've been lacking. Being able concentrate allows you to complete the most basic tasks like thoroughly reading a newspaper article. Although it might not make a huge impact on your life, the ability to focus better on daily things is crucial.

* Focus

The treatment for testosterone replacement will allow you to concentrate even on everyday tasks. Focus issues can be a problem in certain circumstances, like driving, operating machinery or working. Don't let low levels of testosterone to stop you from completing your daily tasks. Focusing better can reduce your time you have to devote to finish an assignment.

* Memory

Memory loss is certainly not enjoyable and it can be difficult to deal with. The thought of forgetting to go to the shop or forgetting your friend's birthday can put yourself in a bind.

Before you were diagnosed as having low levels of testosterone you might have believed you were able to believe that the lack of focus and memory loss was simple results of aging but everyone who is around you will observe how sharper your brain improved after the restoration of the testosterone levels.

It is not possible to lose concentration , and you'll be able to recall more things prior to. One of the greatest benefits associated with testosterone replacement therapy is the results are nearly instantaneous. In just a few weeks of TRT you'll see an improvement in your mental well-being.

4. High-Performance Sex Drive, Performance and Elevated

Discussing your sexual life to anyone, not just your physician, could be embarrassing and uncomfortable.

A low level of testosterone may create unnecessary difficulties in the bedroom , resulting in lower libido, and Erectile dysfunction.

For older males who are older, a lack of sexual drive isn't unusual. However, this doesn't mean that you have to accept it.

As opposed to your younger and more active self, you may be seeing a decline in sexual drive and performance. What's the reason behind this? Males who are aging require an increased level of testosterone than younger males.

Hypogonadism is one the most frequent causes of a decrease in sexual desire. The condition is that causes the body to be insufficiently producing levels of testosterone, which leaves males with a deficiency in sexual desire. The solution to this health issue can be achieved through hormone replacement therapy.

Do not allow the onset of age or any other issue stop you from having fun and enjoying the pleasures of sex. Replacement therapy for testosterone is the most effective treatment for hypogonadism as in any sexual problems.

A decrease in interest in sexual activity won't happen overnight, but it's more of a longer-term issue. Males are more upset as a result of lower libido, than females do. Males are more likely to let this issue affect their lives and cause further difficulties. If you continue to suffer from this issue, you could be disinterested from doing anything that has to do with other people or slip into depression.

Treatment for testosterone replacement will restore the testosterone levels back to normal, thereby stimulating your sexual drive in a healthy way. Studies have shown this therapy significantly improved every aspect of sexual activity. Additionally, research has shown the fact that therapy for testosterone loss has the ability to improve all aspects of sexual activity within few weeks. Men who have been treated with TRT have noticed an increase in sexual drive and orgasm, as well as intercourse satisfaction as well as general satisfaction with sexual activity.

Increase the amount of testosterone back to normal levels will have an immediate impact on your sexual life. You'll notice the benefits of a more sexually active and a greater sexual libido. You and your partner will find that these intimate moments are more fun and fulfilling. You'll definitely feel like you're in the midst of your youth again.

One of the greatest benefits of this therapy for replacement of testosterone is its speed at which results are achieved. Many of the symptoms and signs of low testosterone levels can be eliminated in just a few sessions of the treatment. Some men experienced results almost immediately. They're more focused and their outlook appear to improve in a matter of minutes. Many physical changes can be seen in only several months.

Alongside eliminating the most common symptoms associated with testosterone deficiency the therapy for testosterone replacement also lowers the risk of serious health issues. Anemia, for instance and obesity, diabetes and prostate cancer, as well as osteoporosis and muscle wasting and heart ailments can be prevented and treated using the use of testosterone replacement therapies.

Testosterone replacement therapy actually does provide more than just a cure for man's most insignificant ailments. It improves physical, mental, sexual and emotional health.

Commonly asked Questions (FAQs) regarding Testosterone Replacement Therapy

If you've been diagnosed as having low testosterone, Testosterone Replacement Therapy provides a number of benefits, but there are some dangers.

Here are a few of the most frequently-asked questions regarding TRT:

1. What is the best way to take TRT?

TRT is available in a variety of forms that each have their own advantages and disadvantages.

Subcutaneous pellets - The doctor will place subcutaneous pellets every 3 to six months. Subcutaneous pellets are simple to keep after they are in but they do require minor surgical procedures to treat each dosage.

* Injections - injections are administered two or 10 weeks in between. TRT injections are less expensive when compared to other methods of TRT however they do not give you a steady benefit. Between doses, testosterone levels can drop.

* Buccal patch - each day, you'll place an buccal patch over your gums on the upper. Buccal patches offer comfort, however they can cause gum disease or irritation.

This process involves rubbing gels directly onto your skin each day. Gels are extremely convenient to use, but you should ensure to ensure that nothing is in contact with the area for a while after applying the gel. If they don't, they might get testosterone in their bodies. To eliminate the chance of exposure to others it is recommended to use a nasal gel. It is available for purchase.

* Patches - they are generally very easy to use, however they could cause skin rashes , and could require reapplication during the day.

2. Do I need to stay clear of the testosterone-replacement therapy when suffer from other health issues?

In the opinion of the Endocrine Society, you should not undergo TRT when you suffer with prostate cancer.

There are however, certain studies that suggest that males who have been successfully treated from prostate cancer could undergo TRT provided they are monitored closely for signs of the cancer. Prior to beginning TRT your doctor will assess your likelihood of developing prostate cancer.

It is possible to be advised by a doctor to avoid TRT when you suffer from these conditions that may be more likely to be affected by TRT:

* Over-normal red blood cell count

* Severe congenital heart failure

* Extreme lower urinary tract issues like urinary urgency, or frequency, which are related to benign prostatic hyperplasia (BPH) or an overly large prostate

3. How can I be monitored during my TRT?

In the three or six months following the treatment is started your doctor will check the levels of testosterone. Therefore, you will be tested at least once a year. When your levels of testosterone are normal that is, you'll remain on the current dosage.

When your levels of testosterone are low, your physician may alter the dose. Also your doctor will test the amount of white blood cells.

In the first and two years of TRT Your doctor will examine your bone density , if you suffered from osteoporosis before TRT was first initiated. Your physician will determine your prostate cancer risk when you begin the treatment, and will conduct tests in the 3rd and 6th month. Then, every year.

4. Do testosterone replacement therapies make me feel more energy-filled?

If you're experiencing an insufficient amount of testosterone raising your testosterone levels with testosterone replacement therapy could assist in getting your energy levels to normal. Additionally, TRT may also help revive your sexual drive.

Following the procedure of TRT You may see reduction in body fat as well as an increase in muscle.

5. How long will I have to go through testosterone replacement therapy?

Indefinitely. TRT is not a treatment for testosterone deficiency So your symptoms could be recurred in the event that you discontinue taking it.

6. Are there any risks with the replacement therapy for testosterone?

It is true that TRT can cause side effects, and they could include the following:

* Breasts that are larger

* Testicles shrinkage

* Higher chance of bleeding clots

• Lower number of sperm which can cause an infertility issue.

• Acne, oily and acne-prone skin

7. Is testosterone replacement therapy a treatment for Erectile dysfunction?

If you are suffering from testosterone levels that are low TRT can help increase your sexual drive and improve your ability to get a healthy erection.

The erectile dysfunction, however, can be caused by numerous different reasons. The fact that you have low testosterone levels could not be the sole cause for your Erectile dysfunction. Talk to your doctor to discover what's behind the erectile dysfunction you are experiencing.

The Signs of Testosterone Replacement Therapy is Not appropriate for You

There are many ways of treating testosterone replacement therapy, for example, through gels or patches. They make treating low testosterone levels appear easy, however it's far from being completely free of risk.

There's huge profit by encouraging men to take testosterone supplementation to get an energy boost. Some men may be benefited and feel more energetic and energetic when they supplement their testosterone levels, however the risk of using testosterone replacement therapy could be greater than the benefits in the event that you're not cautious about who receives the treatment.

In actual reality, during a research released within the Journal of the American Medical Association in 2013, a variety of issues were highlighted regarding the dangers associated with replacing testosterone in males. The study surveyed over

1,000 men with low testosterone levels who had undergone coronary angiograms (an exam to determine the severity of coronary heart disease) and who were treated by the treatment of testosterone replacement. Researchers have concluded that the men suffered from a significantly higher risk of suffering a heart attack or stroke than a comparable group of people with low testosterone levels and who had coronary angiography, but weren't subjected to testosterone supplementation.

Many men believe this as the way for coping with exhausted sex and feeling overwhelmed. Most of the time, however these symptoms are normal occurrences in life and the inevitable course of getting older. Testosterone replacement therapy shouldn't be thought of as the source of youngness.

When Testosterone Replacement Therapy Is Not the Answer

The treatment of testosterone replacement has some risks and is therefore not appropriate for everyone. Certain medical conditions and situations make testosterone replacement therapy is a good idea that is worth discussing with a doctor. This includes:

* If you're seriously overweight

Men who weigh 30-40 pounds overweight typically suffer with low testosterone levels. It is not the best reason to seek the testosterone therapy. Losing weight is a far more efficient and healthier alternative.

* If you are suffering from sleep apnea

Sleep apnea that is not treated, can be made worse through treatment with testosterone. Sleep apnea can be described as a condition that causes short, but frequently interruptions in breathing while sleeping that is often accompanied by noises of snoring. If you experience any of the signs of sleep apnea you should have an exam of your sleep in order to establish a correct diagnosis and then try Continuous Positive Airway Pressure (CPAP) or CPAP as a treatment option to treat sleep apnea. If this treatment doesn't help your condition, then it is recommended that you not use testosterone supplementation.

* If you are suffering from polycythemia.

Polycethemia is an illness that causes excessive quantities of blood red cells within your body. The replacement therapy for testosterone may make the condition more severe since testosterone increases the production in red blood cells. This is also an adverse result of the testosterone replacement therapy. Additionally the therapy for testosterone replacement could cause your blood to thicken and increase the chance of having a stroke or heart attacks more likely. If you've had a diagnosis of polycythemia then you should stay clear the testosterone-replacement therapy.

* If you're looking to have children

A young male who would like to have children in the near future must be aware that the use of testosterone replacement therapy can reduce fertility and reduce the number of sperm in his body. If you supplement your testosterone, your brain tends to block the body's natural production of testosterone through the testicles. In addition, when you supplement testosterone, you could see larger muscles, but smaller testicles. The reduction of sperm occurs within 10 weeks after the testosterone-replacement therapy.

* If you suffer from benign prostate disorders

The Endocrine society has also issued a cautionary note about testosterone supplementation in the event that you are experiencing severe urinary tract issues caused by an increased prostate size or if your doctor discovers the presence of a lump on your prostate gland while performing a digital rectal examination. Testosterone can cause the prostate increase in size which can cause signs of benign prostate disease. It is definitely an indication for testosterone replacement therapy, but you should discuss the risks associated with it with your doctor.

* If you suffer from prostate cancer, you should consult your doctor.

The treatment of testosterone replacement therapy doesn't cause prostate cancer. However, it could cause prostate cancer to develop. It's like adding fuel to the fire. As per the guidelines published from the Endocrine Society, you must not use testosterone if you suffer with prostate cancer. If you've been treated successfully for prostate cancer, you may be able undergo testosterone replacement therapy however you must consult with your physician. Although it is very uncommon in males the breast cancer is a significant reason not to take treatment with testosterone.

* If you exhibit the symptoms of low levels testosterone, you are not the only one.

The symptoms and signs of low testosterone could include weak erections decrease in your sex motivation, mood swings and lower energy. A quarter of males supplement with testosterone without getting a blood test. A few symptoms can reveal the exact amount. It is necessary to have testosterone levels that are low that are properly identified by blood tests in conjunction with symptoms to benefit from the treatment.

* If you are only experiencing lower levels of testosterone. The testosterone level of a man decreases naturally after an age threshold of around 40. There is a significant distinction between the normal decline that tends to accelerate when you reach 60 years of age, and the actual levels of testosterone. The testosterone levels can be assessed using an in-

person blood test. But being asymptomatic of low testosterone levels without any indications isn't an adequate reason to seek testosterone replacement treatment.

The negative side effects and risks associated with testosterone replacement therapy might be reasons not to try this therapy or end it if it has already begun. It is important to talk with your doctor. The negative side results of therapy to replace testosterone are acne, skin reactions and breast growth.

If you're able be able to withstand the adverse effects and dangers that come with the use of testosterone replacement therapies your doctor will need to confirm that you are protected from testosterone supplements. A majority of males endure the treatment well and plenty of men benefit from the advantages that it provides, however, you must be on guard. To check the levels of testosterone in your body regularly, blood tests need to be performed.

Keep in mind this: testosterone replacement therapy may not work for certain men.

Common myths about Testosterone Replacement Therapy and the Truth behind them

Most men would like to increase the levels of testosterone in their. When we think about testosterone, we imagine massive muscles and increased sexual performance. However, on the other hand we might also imagine excessive aggression. The reality is that there are numerous myths surrounding testosterone and testosterone replacement treatment. If you're thinking about TRT The following are some of the most common falsehoods, and what is the reality of these myths:

TRT Myth No. 1. You don't need to make the choice to use TRT lightly.

There are many options to treat testosterone, however it is important not to rush into making a decision. Supplementing your testosterone even if you don't require it, or when you purchase it from a pharmacy is a risky choice. It is important to consult your doctor in the process of making a decision. Doctors can provide you with expert opinion.

The decision to embark on major treatment plan is sure to cause a myriad of issues. Talk to your doctor to get accurate and helpful guidance from a professional you can count on.

TRT Myth No. 2. Over-the counter testosterone are suitable alternatives for TRT that are safe.

Men who suffer from erectile dysfunction feel shy about their situation. They don't want to talk about or confess their issues with another person, not even a doctor. The result is that they look for testosterone replacement products that the market products. However, the bad news is these products aren't secure.

Always consult with your physician to confirm that the product you're taking to your body are healthy. Your doctor will also have an idea of the way testosterone could interact with other kinds of medication that you might be taking.

Myths about TRT No.3 The normal levels of testosterone must be viewed as "low"

Certain men's knowledge their "normal" testosterone levels can make them think that the level is "low" testosterone levels. Some men believe they need to increase their levels.

Men typically believe that the increase in testosterone levels is needed to achieve their goals with their partners or develop bigger muscles. However, what these men don't know is that taking excessive amounts of testosterone even though their bodies don't really require it may cause more harm than beneficial. Supplementing with testosterone even when levels are already in the normal range could increase the risk of developing stroke and heart disease, as well as many other serious health issues.

Only after confirmation by a medical professional that you need to undergo TRT is it advisable to consider supplementing with testosterone. It is impossible to determine the cause of this health issue by yourself.

TRT Myth No. 4: Steroids may serve as an alternative to testosterone

Anabolic steroids are synthesized hormones that have a similarity to androgens. Testosterone is regarded as the most powerful androgen However testosterone replacement therapy employs different kinds of steroids than the ones commonly used by bodybuilders. All compounds that simulate hormones constitute steroids. However, there are a few different kinds of steroids that are produced equally or are of medical-grade quality.

TRT Myth No. 5 The testosterone is the same thing as Sperm

No. testosterone is a hormone produced by the testicles . It is responsible to regulate the formation of masculine sexual traits. Testicles perform two main roles: the release of testosterone as well as the generation of, development as well as release of sperm, which occurs in seminiferous tubules.

However the sperm cell is a reproductive cell, also known as a male gamete whose growth is influenced by the change of testosterone-producing hormones. Sperm can impotently infect females, while testosterone can simply make her feel uncomfortable and hot.

TRT Myth No. 3. Excessive levels of testosterone can cause you to become more aggressive

Yes. In excess levels of testosterone in your body may result in your hairline beginning to reced and the testicles to shrink and even your mood to change often.

Do you know if there are any differences in Testosterone Replacement Therapy (TRT) and Human Growth Hormone (HGH)?

Testosterone as well as human growth hormone (HGH) are two kinds of anabolic steroids that are commonly used by bodybuilders to increase their body mass. HGH and testosterone have both legitimate medical benefits, however they are most commonly referred to for their use as supplements to build muscle. Although both have the same purpose however, they are distinct compounds.

Testosterone is the name of a hormone that is produced naturally by males and females. However men are more likely to produce testosterone than women. The testosterone form utilized by bodybuilders is synthetic and synthesized in a lab. Testosterone triggers the body to produce more muscle mass and reduce body fat, making it an ideal choice for bodybuilders of all types. It is usually used alongside other forms of steroids for anabolic use by the majority of bodybuilders as they give incredible results when combined together.

Most bodybuilders use testosterone during cycles. This is because testosterone tends to reduce the body's natural testosterone production The cycle of testosterone can prevent a permanent shutdown. The typical testosterone cycle for bodybuilders consists of around eight weeks of supplementation with steroids then a 4 week post-cycle treatment. Testosterone supplements can be found in a variety of forms, including pills, injections, creams and patches. Bodybuilders generally opt with testosterone shots. It is most effective method. The the majority of chemical compounds have to be injected every other week.

The hormone that is produced by the human body is also synthesized naturally by the body. Human growth hormone is made by the pituitary gland in order to regulate the growth process in the early years of childhood. Bodybuilders make use of a synthetic form of this hormone because it is able to heal injured tissues and aid in the growth of lean muscle mass. Human growth hormone causes organs and bones to expand when used in large quantities, which keeps a lot of people from using it.

Are there any adverse consequences from HGH?

Water retention is one of the most frequent side effect of HGH and some people holding up to 5 lbs of weight in water. Carpal tunnels can also happen but usually they disappear after some weeks.

Like the testosterone-replacement therapy used by bodybuilders, they typically utilize human growth hormone cycles for a time of 6-8 weeks, and injecting 5 to 7 times one week. In this time, bodybuilders are likely to gain more muscle mass and strength , while getting rid of fat. When using one HGH cycle, it's typical to gain 10-20 kg of mass.

Chapter 9: What Testosterone Is Vital?

Men and boys?

Testosterone triggers the physical changes that turn the boy into an adult. This stage of the life span is known as Adolescence. The changes include

Penis growth and the testes

The growth of pubic, facial and body hair

Amplification of the voice

Muscles and bones are built by building strong bones and muscles.

Growing more taller

Men also require normal levels of this hormone in order to produce Sperm and are able to produce children.

How does testosterone work?

The pituitary and brain located in the middle of our brains, manage the testosterone production through tests. From there, testosterone moves through your bloodstream to perform its job.

The levels of testosterone fluctuate depending on the time of the day. They tend to be the highest in the morning and lower in the evening.

Testosterone levels are the most notable at ages 20-30 and then gradually decrease from age 30 to 35.

What is the worst thing that can happen when testosterone levels are high?

There are many reasons why testosterone levels can drop and remain low. In less cases testosterone levels may be excessive. When testosterone levels are not in the right place, health problems can occur. Find out if you should have your testosterone level tested for any of the conditions that are listed below. Treatment is a possibility to resolve hormone issues.

Low testosterone

The first signs (transforms the sensation you experience) and indications (abnormalities which your doctor finds) that indicate low testosterone levels in men are

A drop in the sex can

Poor erections

Low Sperm Tally

Breasts that are weak or large

In the future, testosterone levels can cause a decline in bone and muscle quality, as well as less vitality as well as lower fertility.

Certain things may lower testosterone levels such as excessive exercise, inadequate nutrition, or a genuine illness. Maintaining a healthy lifestyle through regular exercise and a good diet can maintain normal testosterone levels.

High testosterone

When young men are able to produce too much testosterone, they may be prone to pubescence young (before the age of 9). A few rare diseases such as specific types of tumors can cause men to produce testosterone earlier than normal.

Young men can also get too much testosterone when they come in contact with the testosterone gel that a mature man is using to treat.

How do you determine you are getting in terms of your level of testosterone?

To quantify your testosterone level, your specialist can arrange a blood test. The test must be performed in the early morning, between 7:15 to 10:00. If the result isn't typical, it is recommended to repeat the test in order to be sure that there is no doubt about the result. For healthy men testosterone levels may fluctuate dramatically from day to day tests, and therefore a follow-up test may be normal.

How to increase Testosterone levels naturally

We've finally reached the last article of Testosterone Week and in view of the feedback from everyone it's the one you've been looking most for. Today I'll be sharing the things I learned during my 90-day study in order to double my free testosterone and aggregate levels.

I'm worried that I don't have any awesome "privileged knowledge" to share, and there's no easy alternative methods to boost your testosterone. If you're expecting something different from a supplement or mix or other body-hack that can immediately and effectively boost your testosterone levels, then what follows will surely fall short. Contrary to what a handful of websites or organizations might claim, there's no one thing that can boost your testosterone over long-term.

The fact can be that increasing your testosterone usually is a matter of making some modifications to your eating habits and your lifestyle. You'll discover that the things I did to boost T to a large extent came from eating more nutritious food and exercising more effectively and getting more rest. This is all there is. As like most aspects of life, unnoticed particulars are the biggest problem and I'll tell you exactly what I did and provide a look-up what I did to explain how the things I did helped me increase my testosterone levels.

The good news is that, while the items I've suggested below will boost your testosterone levels, their effect isn't just limited to testosterone. They'll dramatically improve overall health and wellbeing as well.

What are your options to Replace Your Equipment?

If you're a man who is suffers from side effects, such as such as a decreased sex drive, erectile dysfunction or a disengaged mind-set as well as problems with memory and fixation and suspect low testosterone could be at your fault, you should test your testosterone levels. Since testosterone levels are erratic throughout your daytime, it's likely require more than just one blood test to get the most accurate information about your testosterone levels.

If your levels are in the low range, then there's many bio-identical and synthetic testosterone supplements available, additionally DHEA is the largest androgen precursor prohormone that is found in our body. This implies this is actually the most base material that your body uses to make other essential hormones which include testosterone in males and estrogen in women.

I would suggest the use of bio-identical hormones and then under the supervision of a holistic doctor who can track the levels of your hormones to determine if you need supplements.

It is true that prior to deciding on this route there are numerous methods you can try to improve the testosterone levels of your normal. They are appropriate to all purposes and for any person, since they offer the most important "symptoms."

1. Simply lose weight

If you're overweight, losing weight can boost the amount of testosterone in your body, according to the study presented at the Endocrine Society's meeting in 2012. Men who are overweight will likely have lower testosterone levels at the beginning This is an important way to boost your body's production of testosterone at the time you require it most.

If you're serious in your quest to lose weight then you should be sure to limit the amount of sugar prepared into your daily diet, because evidence is mounting that the abundance of sugar, particularly fructose is the main driver of the epidemic of obesity. Therefore, removing the consumption of pop out of your diet is crucial as is limiting fructose that is found in processed foods and juices of fruit, as well as in unnatural fruit , and the purportedly "healthy" sweeteners such as agave.

In a perfect world , you must keep your overall fructose consumption to less than 25 grams per day, and that includes fruits. This is particularly true when you suffer from insulin resistance, are overweight, suffer from diabetes, hypertension or high cholesterol.

In addition to removing or limiting the amount of fructose you consume, it is crucial to remove all grains and eliminate any toxins (even the most basic) of your diet. Milk is a source of sugar known as lactose. It has been found to raise insulin resistance, so it is recommended to stay away from it if trying to lose weight.

The refined starches such as breakfast oats bagels, waffles and bagels pretzels, and many other foods prepared for consumption also quickly break down into sugar, raise your insulin levels and can cause insulin resistance which is the principal underlying component of almost every health condition and disease that is not known as weight gain.

When you eliminate these unhealthy foods out of your meals it is essential to replace them with nutritious alternatives such as fruits and vegetables, as well as healthy fats (including regular saturated fats!). Your body will gravitate towards the micronutrients in thick vegetables over sugars or grains because they ease back the transition to glucose and other sugars and decreases your insulin levels. If you eliminate sugar and grains from your dinners, you must drastically increase the amount of vegetables you consume and be sure you're eating the right amount of protein and healthy fats often.

I've put together a point-by-point controlled guideline for this kind of healthy diet program within my comprehensive nutrition plan I'm asking that you consult with this guideline in your efforts to slim down.

Your diet are the primary factor in achieving your weight loss goals - intense, short-burst type exercises, like the Peak Fitness Program, a every week, in conjunction with a complete fitness plan is crucial and offers an added advantage.

2. High-Intensity Training such as Peak Fitness (Especially Combined with Intermittent Fasting)

The intermittent fasting as well as short intense exercises have been proven to increase testosterone levels.

It is not the same as the intensity of exercise or the delay in moderate exercise. Both have been proven to have negative or no effect upon testosterone levels.

The intermittent increase in speed that makes it possible to accelerate the flow of hormones that promote satiety, such as leptin, insulin, Adiponectin (adiponectin), glucagon-like- (GLP-1) and colecystokinin (CKK) and melanocortins each of them as testosterone-related activities that are not healthy boost moxie levels and prevent the decline in testosterone due to age.

Having a whey protein supper after exercise can further improve the satiety/testosterone-boosting sway (hunger hormones cause the opposite impact on your testosterone and charisma). Here's a brief overview of what a typical high intensity Peak Fitness routine may resemble:

Get ready for three minutes of warm-up.

Try to be as stiff as you are able for thirty minutes. You should feel as if you can't ever in any manner, form or form, continue for a couple of minutes.

You can recover at a medium or rapid pace for about 90 seconds.

Repeat the high-intensity exercise and recovery seven more times.

It's not difficult to see that the whole exercise is only 20 minutes. 20 minutes! This is truly a wonderful thing. Within the 20 minutes 75 percent of the time is spent warming up, recovering , or cooling down. It's really just working in a gruelling only four minutes. It's hard to believe even if you've never attempted this before that you could reap the benefits of the four minutes you exercising. This is it.

Be aware that you are able to use to the greatest extent all the equipment that you require to accomplish this, such as such as a curving machine, treadmill, swimming in spite of running outside (despite knowing that you must be careful to keep an appropriate distance from injuries) Insofar as you're exerting yourself as hard to the limit for the duration of 30 minutes. Whatever you choose to do, ensure that you extend your body appropriately and gradually increase your pace to avoid injuries. Start with a few reps before moving up to more and don't try to complete each of the eight repetitions on the first time you try this, especially if you haven't been doing it for a while.

There is more information on this subject in an earlier article written about intermittent fasting.

3. Spend a lot of Zinc

Zinc is a vital mineral for the generation of testosterone. the addition of zinc supplements to your diet for as little as six weeks is proven to cause a measurable rise in testosterone in men who have low levels.1 Additionally, research has discovered that reducing the intake of zinc can trigger a dramatic reduction in testosterone levels, whereas zinc supplementation can increase it2 - and can even protect men from the effects of exercise on testosterone levels.3

It's estimated that as high as 45 percent of adulthood-aged adults who are over 60 could have lower than the recommended daily intake of zinc. regardless of whether supplements from dietary sources were considered, 20-25 percent of the more experienced adulthood had insufficient zinc intakes as determined by an National Health and Nutrition Examination Survey.

Your diet is the greatest source of zinc. Alongside proteins-rich foods such as fish and meats, other good sources of zinc are crude cheese, crude milk beans, yogurt, or kefir that is made with crude milk. It isn't easy to get enough zinc in your diet for those who love vegetables and meat-eaters as well, to a large degree due to traditional farming practices that rely heavily on pesticides and composts of substances. Chemicals drain the soil of supplements ... nutrients such as zinc that are consumed by plants, and then transferred to you.

In many instances it is possible to further deplete the nutrition in your food due to the way you prepare the food. In the majority of meals, cooking will certainly reduce the levels of nutrients like zinc ... especially if you over-cook it as many do.

If you decide to take zinc supplements, you should stick to a dose less than 40 mg per day that is the maximum amount recommended for adults. In excess, zinc may hinder your body's ability to absorb other minerals, including copper, and could cause a queasiness reaction.

4. Strength Training

Alongside Peak Fitness, quality training is also known as testosterone levels, provided you're working out hard enough. When you are training is required to boost testosterone levels is required, you'll need to raise the weight and decrease your number of reps. And then focus on exercises that target multiple muscles, like dead lifting or squats.

It is possible to "turbo-charge" your weight training by slowing down your pace. By slowing your pace is changing it into a vigorous exercise. A slow, steady movement allows your muscles, on an tiny level, to be able to get to the highest amount of cross-scaffolds that connect the protein filaments that cause movements in the muscles.

5. Improve your Vitamin D Levels

Vitamin D is an steroid hormone, is vital for the proper development of the cells that make up the sperm and also helps maintain semen quality and the sperm tally. Vitamin D can also increase levels of testosterone which may help Moxie. In one study, obese people who took vitamin D supplements showed significant increases of testosterone after one year.5

Vitamin D deficiency is currently at epidemic levels across the United States and many other regions around the world to a large extent because people aren't investing enough energy in the sun to aid the vital process for the process of vitamin D creation.

The first step to making sure you're receiving all the advantages from vitamin D is to figure out what your levels are by taking the 25(OH)D test, also known as 25-hydroxyvitamin D.

A few years ago the recommended dosage was 40-60 nanograms per milliliter (ng/ml) but in the case lately, the recommended vitamin D levels have been elevated to 50 to 70 mg/ml.

For bringing your levels to the proper range that you need, sun exposure is the most effective method to increase the levels of vitamin D; exposure to a large portion of your skin to the most light shades of pink or as close to a sun-powered twelve as you can it is usually necessary to achieve sufficient vitamin D production. If sun exposure isn't possible then a tanning bed that is sheltered (with electronic stabilizers instead of beautiful counterweights to keep clear of unnecessary exposure for EMF fields) can be used.

If nothing else works the vitamin D3 supplement could be taken orally. However, researchers suggest that grown-ups have the needs to consume 8,000 IU of vitamin D each day, keeping in mind the aim of bringing their levels to above 40 ng/ml. This is the absolute minimum requirement to prevent disease.

6. Lessen Stress

If you're in a large amount in stress or tension, your body produces an abnormal amount of cortisol, a stress hormone. The hormone blocks testosterone's effects, due to the fact that from a physiological perspective, testosterone-related behaviors (mating and fighting and animosity) could have lowered your chances of survival an emergency (subsequently in you'll experience the "battle or flee" reaction takes over and cortisol's cordiality is a major factor).

In today's the world, constant stress and therefore elevated levels of cortisol could indicate that testosterone's properties are impeded over the long term and that's why you must keep your distance from.

My most effective overall method to reduce anxiety to manage stress is EFT (Emotional Freedom Technique) that is similar to acupuncture but without needles. It's a simple, non-cost tool to release psychological burden quickly and easily and is so natural that even children can master it. Other tools for stress reduction that are regular and have a an excellent success rate include the supplication of God and God, yoga, meditation, and giggling for instance. Learning helps to relax the mind like deep breathing and positive visualisation, that are considered to be an example of the "language" for the subliminal.

If you create an image of what you'd love to experience your brain will recognize and start to assist you in making the needed biological and neurological adjustments.

7. Eliminate or limit the amount of sugar in Your diet

Testosterone levels drop when you consume sugar, which could be because of the fact that sugar triggers a higher insulin level, which is another factor that causes lower levels of testosterone.7

When we take into consideration USDA appraisals, the typical American consumes about the equivalent of 12 teaspoons sugar per day, which is approximately 2 tons of sugar in the course of their lives.

The reason we consume this amount of sugar isn't difficult to comprehend - it is delicious, and makes us happy by stimulating an inherent process that occurs in your brain via the transmission of opioid and dopamine signals.

What it's doing to us both on the physical and emotional level is a different story completely and the majority of people are able to see real improvement in their health and wellbeing by restricting or completely eliminating sugar in their weight-loss strategies. Be aware of foods that are laden with fructose and sugar, and grains such as pasta and bread ought to be a minimum.

If you're suffering from sugar dependence and are having trouble managing cravings, I highly recommend taking a look at a vitality brain research technique known as Turbo Tapping, which has provided numerous "soda addicts" overcome their cravings for sweets and will help you satisfy any sweet craving that you may have.

8. Eat Healthily Fats

Healthy means not just monounsaturated and polyunsaturated oils like those found in nuts and avocados however, they are also saturated since they are crucial in building testosterone. Studies have shown that a diet regimen that has less than 40 percent of energy as fat (and mostly comes from animal sources, i.e. submerged) result in a decrease in testosterone levels.8

My personal eating habits are between 60 and 70 percent healthy fats, and experts agree that the best diet is somewhere between 50 and 70 percent fat.

It is essential to know that your body needs to soak fats from vegetable and animal source, (for examples, such as meat dairy, dairy products, specific oils and tropical plants like coconut) for optimal functioning and, if you ignore this essential nutritional category for sugar, grains , and other carbs that are boring that are not healthy for you, your weight and health will be able to last. Examples of healthy fats that which you can consume a larger quantity of to boost your testosterone levels a boost are:

Olive oil and olives

Coconut oil and coconuts

Raw nuts include, for instance pecans, almonds, or pecans

Butter made from grass-fed natural milk

Avocados

Organic eggs from pastures

The meats of the grass are encouraged to graze

Palm oil

Natural nut oils that are not heated

9. Improve your intake of Branch Chain Amino acids (BCAA) through foods such as Whey Protein

Research suggests that BCAAs increase testosterone levels, particularly when they are combined with resistance training.9 Although BCAAs can be found through supplement structures there are astonishing convergences of BCAAs, like leucine, in dairy products - specifically top quality cheeses and whey proteins.

Although you may get leucine from your usual food supply, it's typically wasted or used as a building obstruction instead of being an anabolic operator. To create the ideal atmosphere for anabolic, you need to increase the amount of leucine you use beyond the normal maintenance levels.

Remember that using leucine to free shape amino corrosive is very harmful. When amino acids from the free frame are administered in a controlled manner and then get into your system, interfering with insulin production and affecting the body's control of glycemic. Sustenance-based leucine is the ideal shape to aid your muscles and not cause any discomfort.

Testosterone therapy

If you are suffering from anxiety with high or low testosterone levels, a physician could run a blood test in order to measure the level of testosterone in the blood of the patient. When doctors detect low testosterone, they may suggest testosterone therapy, which the patient is given an artificial form of testosterone. It is available through the following forms A gel that can be attached to the upper arms and shoulders or abdomen, every day; a patch of skin applied to your body, or the scrotum for two times each day; a solution that is attached to the armpit; injections once several weeks; a patch placed on the gums at least twice a each day; or inserts that last between 4 and 6 months.

The users of testosterone gels should be aware of safety precautions, such as washing their hands and covering areas that the gel is attached according to the U.S. food and Drug Administration. Younger and females should not touch the gel or skin on which the fix or gel is connected.

In older, more experienced men suffering from real testosterone deficiencies The treatment of testosterone has been proven to boost the quality of their sex drives experts claim.

It's true sometimes, the adverse effects of erectile dysfunction can be caused by other ailments such as diabetes and depression according to Mayo Clinic. The treatment of the men affected with testosterone hormones won't improve the symptoms.

As a result the treatment of testosterone can lower the sperm count, and Michael A. Werner, an expert in andropause also known as "male menopausal,"" suggests that men who wish to have a to have a future pregnancy keep a separation from testosterone treatments. Other side effects include a higher chances of developing heart problems for older men who have mobility issues, as per an article published by Boston Medical Center. The treatment may raise the chance of developing rest apnea, accelerate bosom and prostate growth, and may even lead to the growth of prostate tumors as per reports from the Mayo Clinic.

Things Testosterone Can Do to Your Body

You hear "testosterone" as well, and then the first thing you might think of is anger. However, new research by Bonn University University of Bonn shows that the commonly misunderstood hormone could promote the behavior of a person and allow for legitimate interactions.

Specialists administered 46 people testosterone gel, and 45 others who received a fake treatment. The next day, each of the 91 participants were asked to roll the ivory in private, record the numbers they scored and receive cash depending on their results--with those who had the best results earning more cash. After paying the participants, the researchers discovered that those who received testosterone gel reported their numbers more honestly.

The reason is that high levels of testosterone boost your self-esteem and help you build your mental picture. But cheating puts both of you in danger, according to experts. With just a few dollars hanging around there was no reason for the participants to risk it all.

It's true testosterone can do more than just keeping you legal. Researchers have discovered that testosterone does not only let testosterone affect the way you behave, but also the way you conduct yourself can impact the levels of testosterone, too. Here are some more crazy things testosterone can provide help with.

Get the Girl

Researchers of Wayne State University contrasted two groups of men who were competing to winning the attention of attractive women and discovered that those who had lower testosterone levels didn't have in the way of winning. Men with the highest testosterone levels were more confident and controlled the conversation and bonded better with women.

Avoid an untimely Death

What could "T" help you? The first thing to consider is delay your meeting with the soul-sharper? Low testosterone levels have been connected to type 2 obesity and diabetes. Furthermore it has been proven by a handful of studies that have proven that those who have lower levels are at an increased risk of developing coronary disease.

Help her with getting off

Testosterone can benefit women in a significant way. According to a report by the University of Michigan, women who have higher levels of T-hormone are more likely to have positive sexual encounters. Researchers found that women who have high levels of testosterone perceived sex as soothing calm, relaxing and peaceful. Previous studies have also revealed that women with higher levels of testosterone have more sexual pleasure and may even reach their an emotional climax. Score.

Involve yourself in sexual relationships in Sync

Did you know that your body's T-levels are matched in relation to menstrual cycles? In a study released in the journal Hormones & Behavior researchers discovered that testosterone levels peak every 28 days. It also occurs on weekends, which is the time when men are reported to have the most sexual experience. Also, having sexual contact with new or multiple partners can cause your testosterone levels to rise in accordance with the research.

Be an Optimist

People who watched porn experienced an increase of 35 percent in testosterone between an hour and a quarter in the aftermath of watching the show, as per research published in The Archives of Sexual Behavior. They were absolutely thrilled by the experience. After watching the hypnotic recordings the men noticed a greater level of energy and enthusiasm. (We can see the reasons right now: "Yet it perks me up, sweet nectar!")

Can cause a Financial Crisis

Researchers examined 98 men to determine their testosterone levels and willingness to risk it all in the form of a PC simulation. The results: Men who had higher testosterone levels were more likely to put more money into their savings. Therefore, would we be able of blame testosterone for the decrease in testosterone?

The benefits of Testosterone

Testosterone is a hormone which is created primarily by the testicles. It plays a crucial role in the masculine characteristics and male growth. The testosterone production crests in the pre-adulthood period and in the beginning of adulthood. Following that, it's normal for levels to decrease little by little each year.

Testosterone plays a significant role in the development of solid bones and bulk. It is also responsible for males' powerful voices. It also can also influence sex drives. In men, low testosterone levels male are known as hypogonadism.

Women also have testosterone but in smaller quantities. For women, the adrenal glands and ovaries make testosterone.

1. A healthy heart and blood

A healthy heart pump blood to the rest of the body. It supplies organs and muscles with the oxygen needed for peak performance.

Low levels of testosterone are connected to a myriad of cardiovascular risk. As per Harvard Medical School, testosterone replacement therapy can increase the coronary veins. This could be beneficial for people suffering from angina, mid-section pain and weight gain when your heart isn't getting enough blood.

Testosterone may also cause blood platelet counts to rise in a way that is to be thankful for in the event of fragility (low number of red blood cells).

2. Letting go of fat and gaining muscle

Leaner body mass reduces the weight and boosts vitality. There is some evidence to suggest that testosterone treatments can reduce the amount of fat in your body and improve the strength and size of your muscles. The effect is stronger when combined with high-quality training and exercises.

A study of 108 men older than 65 found that treatment with testosterone dramatically reduced fat, especially in the legs and arms. These same men experienced an increase in the mass of incline typically within the compartment for storage. The patients received testosterone treatment for 36-months.

3. Stronger Bones

Solid bones support your muscles and organs that can aid in the performance of your athletes. As we age, testosterone levels decrease, so does bone density decreases. This increases the risk of having weak bone and the development of osteoporosis. An article published in the Journal of Clinical Endocrinology and Metabolism suggests that older men may boost their bone density through the therapy of testosterone replacement. This is especially true for those who had low levels of testosterone prior to starting treatment.

4. Better Libido

Testosterone levels usually increase with sexual activity and excitement. Testosterone levels drop off after long periods of absence. Additionally, higher levels of testosterone can trigger sexual desire and continues the cycle. Testosterone is known to have a positive effect on a man's sexual desire and performance.

Testosterone can also affect the woman's sexual drive. As per the Mayo Clinic, there aren't many information about long-term health in women, therefore experts might be cautious before they prescribe the hormone.

5. Mood Enhance Mood

Testosterone levels usually increase with the excitement of sexual activity and. They fall during long periods of abstinence. Additionally, increased testosterone stimulates sexual desire and continues the cycle. Based on research from Harvard Medical School, testosterone can positively impact the sexual desire of men and performance.

Testosterone is also a factor in women's sexual drive. Based on the Mayo Clinic, there aren't many studies on long-term security for women, therefore experts might not be sure to endorse the practice.

6. Testosterone enhances charisma and the erections.

Testosterone is a hormone that can be used to enhance sexual desire which is why it's not surprising that breaking of the erectile tract are among the most common indicators of low testosterone that men look for. If you've noticed a sudden slowing of your enthusiasm for sexual activity, it could be due to low testosterone.

If I mentioned to people that I was undertaking an experiment to boost my testosterone levels, the question that I would hear from people in a quiet voice was "Along this line did it improve your sexual relationships?" In truth, I didn't notice any changes. I was able to enjoy a wholesome and healthy sexual relationship prior to the experiment, and continued to be a good co-sex person for a brief period of time after. I think I was a little runny than I had hoped, but not much. If you'd been struggling with low T for time and decided to boost it, you'd be seeing improvement in the room department.

Testosterone may reduce your risk of getting Alzheimer's disease.

A handful of studies have found that low testosterone levels are linked to a greater risk of developing Alzheimer's disease. In a recent study published by researchers at the University of Hong Kong, researchers looked at the case of 153 Chinese individuals who were recruited from various social areas. They were 55 years old or more living with their families, and did not suffer from dementia. The majority of them were found to have mild cognitive impairmentthat is, issues with clarity of thought and memory issues.

Within one year, 10 males who were part of the cognitively impaired group developed possible Alzheimer's disease. The men have also been found to be deficient in testosterone levels in the body's tissues.

The study isn't just one of many. Specialists from the University of Southern California have found that an increase in hormone levels among mice suffering from Alzheimer's actually slows the progression in the course of this disease. This idea has led scientists to propose that maintaining the ideal levels of testosterone throughout the aging process could help prevent the disease from spreading to humans.

8. Testosterone could improve cognitive performance.

The research has demonstrated the link to T-levels and cognitive capacity, particularly among older men. A study conducted by Dutch researchers found an immediate linear connection between the T levels and cognitive performance, whereas studies have also found that there is a linear connection between memory misfortunes and levels of testosterone. Because of these findings, many researchers believe that testosterone plays a role in preventing the deterioration of brain tissue in men who are aging. The association between the hormone and cognition is the reason for a lot of the negative effects associated with testosterone levels in men are confusion, memory problems, trouble concentration, as well as "fogginess."

Although studies haven't discovered an association between the levels of testosterone with cognitive capacity in younger people, that isn't going to stop you from aiming to achieve the ideal levels of testosterone. It is essential to establish healthy testosterone practices now so that you'll be able to benefit from your senior years.

9. Testosterone may increase your the level of competition.

Men are not known as to be a team player and testosterone could be to be the driver behind our desire to beat the competition. Testosterone is connected to a man's desire for strength as well as standing (Dabbs as well as Dabbs 2000). Testosterone increases prior to an event or battle - creating consequences for hemoglobin and bulk, speeding up reactions, increasing vision, and enhancing your sense of determination and determination. Also, it increases the level of "gameness:" One study revealed that a man's testosterone levels after losing a diversion was a predictor of how likely he would be back for a second round. People who experienced a dramatic drop in their testosterone levels were less likely to participate in a second round, whereas those who had very little or no change in levels of testosterone were more involved in the game. The researchers concluded with the impression that T is among the factors that drive competitiveness in males.

Side Effects and potential risks

Some of the symptoms of testosterone therapy include swelling of the skin, liquid maintenance, and more frequent urine production. The less common symptoms are the enlargement of the bosom and a decrease in testicular size.

Treatments for medicine testosterone are available in the form of gels, patches for skin and intramuscular injections. Each can trigger signs and symptoms. If you are applying gels, be cautious not to substitute the gel with other gels. The patches can cause irritation to the skin. Intramuscular injections can cause emotional reactions.

Treatment with testosterone is not recommended for people suffering from bosom or prostate growth. If you are older the testosterone treatment may decrease the rest apnea. Treatment with testosterone may reduce the number of sperm and also increase the forcefulness of methods.

The truth of the matter is that therapy with testosterone may cause a variety of health issues that aren't justifiable regardless of the advantages. Additionally, men aren't always the only ones affected by these medications. Children, women as well as pets are adversely affected.

Some men are making lawsuits against the manufacturers of testosterone products, claiming they concealed the risks of their products.

The use of testosterone therapy and heart Attacks

A few studies documented a few conceivable risks for men taking testosterone-enhancing drugs. These drugs can be linked to several heart-related issues and heart attacks.

One of the most notable studies, released on the 29th of January 2014 within the PLoS One diary, observed that older men than 65 years old and younger people with no known coronary disease were twice as likely to experiencing a heart attack after the first ninety days of testosterone treatment.

The study involved 56,000 patients , and was conducted by National Cancer Institute and UCLA. The researchers looked into the data of patients prior to and after they were given their first testosterone solution.

The 2014 study is not the only one to call for concerns about cardiovascular risks related to testosterone replacement medications.

In the years 2010 and 2013, researchers supervised two studies that were published in the New England Journal of Medicine (NEJM) as well as The Journal of the American Medical Association (JAMA) separately. The research involved people who were weak or old and revealed that those who are vulnerable or elderly will likely suffer the negative effects of several heart "events," including heart attacks.

Truth is, during the NEJM study, one person was thrown out of the pool and researchers believed it was an assault on the heart that was caused through testosterone use.

Conclusion

Testosterone boosters can boost the testosterone levels, but that should be clear from the title of this specific kind of supplement for games. Although some are more effective in comparison to others. boosters are designed to enhance the capacity of your body to make more testosterone than normal. They're not meant to replace the testosterone you already have in any way, but rather to increase your ability to produce a higher amount of this important hormone.

As it happens how much could you expect to experience by boosting your levels of T-support? What can a quality T-supporter to accomplish for you? Fantastic questions! In this useful guide I'll explain the purpose of T-boosters and the benefits you can expect from using them.

Testosterone makes you more grounded. There are a variety of mechanisms at work of this, ranging from the increased dimensions of the muscles, giving a greater favorable effects to an increase in resistance in the center of the recreation. The most important issue is that the same amount of steroid-taking baseball players, football players as well as sprinters, hurlers, and weightlifters will inform you that that more testosterone equals better quality. If you're solid, you are able to lift heavier weights that bring more bulk. This means you'll be able to lift heavier weights and feel more secure... as the list goes on. In contrast, when steroids increase your testosterone levels normally the T-promoter allows your body to generate more testosterone normal testosterone levels - this is a major distinction.

If you want to build muscles, you must increase your testosterone levels. And If your testosterone levels are high and you are able to see gains in muscle that are less challenging. Even though it is true that you will not be as thrilling as those who take one gram of steroids per week, you will experience a steady, moderate and steady increase in the size of your muscles after using a testosterone booster. This growth in muscle mass comes alongside an improvement in quality. Because steroids cause such an immediate increase in the size of muscles It is not uncommon to see clients, as they get off the rig, to lose a

183

large amount of the muscles they gained. This shouldn't be the case with testosterone boosters. If you're training regularly and eat a healthy diet and eat properly, the muscle that you gain using a high-quality T-promoter should to be kept.